All of us are drug users, in the broadest sense of the word. Drugs can be medicines, they can be used for pleasure, and they can also be used to protect our long-term health. It is important that we are well informed about the drugs we use – how they work, their benefits, and their risks. This book is a unique guide for the general science reader to the drugs of everyday life – from the main types of medicine through to recreational drugs and food supplements. It looks at how drugs interact with their targets in the body, where they come from, how they are developed and what drugs to expect in the future. All the major pharmaceutical medicines are reviewed – painkillers, antibiotics, anti-cancer drugs, anti-depressants, heart drugs, tranquillisers and hormones. However this book is much more than a consumer handbook – it also conveys the fascinating science of drug discovery in an easily accessible way.

Susan Aldridge is a professional science writer and medical editor for *Focus* magazine, having been a research scientist. She is a Fellow of the Royal Society of Medicine.

SUSAN ALDRIDGE

Magic Molecules

how drugs work

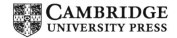

CAMBRIDGE
UNIVERSITY PRESS

CAMBRIDGE UNIVERSITY PRESS
Cambridge, New York, Melbourne, Madrid, Cape Town, Singapore, São Paulo

Cambridge University Press
The Edinburgh Building, Cambridge CB2 8RU, UK

Published in the United States of America by Cambridge University Press, New York

www.cambridge.org
Information on this title: www.cambridge.org/9780521584142

First published 1998
This digitally printed version 2007

A catalogue record for this publication is available from the British Library

Library of Congress Cataloguing in Publication data

Aldridge, Susan.
    Magic Molecules : how drugs work / Susan Aldridge.
        p.   cm.
    ISBN 0 521 58414 0 (hb)
    1. Drugs–Mechanism of action–Popular works.   I. Title.
    RM301.15.A43   1998
    615'.7—dc21   98–21346 CIP

ISBN 978-0-521-58414-2 hardback
ISBN 978-0-521-04415-8 paperback

Every effort has been made in preparing this book to provide accurate and up-to-date information which is in accord with accepted standards and practice at the time of publication. Although case histories are drawn from actual cases, every effort has been made to disguise the identities of the individuals involved. Nevertheless, the authors, editors and publishers can make no warranties that the information contained herein is totally free from error, not least because clinical standards are constantly changing through research and regulation. The authors, editors and publishers therefore disclaim all liability for direct or consequential damages resulting from the use of material contained in this book. Readers are strongly advised to pay careful attention to information provided by the manufacturer of any drugs or equipment that they plan to use.

Contents

Illustrations

Acknowledgements

I am grateful to the following people for the help they have given me with the preparation of this book: Nick Henderson and Dr Gordon Fryers of the European Aspirin Foundation, Dr Mike Stillings of Reckitt and Colman, Bill Kirkness from the Association of the British Pharmaceutical Industry, Shaida Dorabjee of the Centre for Medicines Research, Katy Griggs of the British Diabetic Association, Philip Connolly and Corinne Gordon of Glaxo Wellcome, and library staff at the Institute for the Study of Drug Dependence.

I would also like to thank the editors at Cambridge University Press who have been involved in this book, in particular Tim Benton for his support at the outset of the project, and Barnaby Willitts for his comments on the manuscript.

Introduction

Drugs have an impact on all our lives. Many people rely on a daily dose of aspirin or insulin to maintain their long-term health. Others may hope for better drugs to treat challenging illnesses such as cancer or schizophrenia. Away from the realm of serious disease, casual use of painkillers or indigestion remedies relieves minor aches and pains. And most people use some form of recreational drug such as caffeine, alcohol, or nicotine to help them cope with the stresses and strains of everyday life – or just for pleasure.

New drugs are coming onto the market all the time. There are now effective treatments for stroke, AIDS, and multiple sclerosis – where none existed before. Prescribing habits change too – long-term use of tranquillisers and sleeping pills is now frowned on, and slimming drugs are, officially, off limits. The range of medicines available over the counter is continually changing too. Now you can buy the anti-ulcer drug Zantac without a prescription, but some hay-fever remedies and even paracetamol (in large quantities) have moved into the prescription only category. Walk into a health food shop and you will discover an alternative pharmacy – vitamins, minerals, phytochemicals and herbs – in a bewildering array of strengths and dosages.

But how well do we understand the drugs we are prescribed or choose to take? What informs our doctor's choices, and our own? And is there really a 'pill for every ill'? Where *do* you find out about the drugs you take?

By law, companies must insert an information leaflet into every packet of a prescription drug. While efforts have been made recently to make these more comprehensible and accessible, they say far more about side effects and contraindications than they do about whether, why, and how the drug might improve the consumer's quality of life. And an information leaflet cannot even hint at the fascination of the science that lies behind the drug.

Turn to the media and there is certainly no lack of drama when it comes to discussing drugs. Television and newspapers tend to concentrate on new 'wonder' drugs (in reality, there is no such thing). For instance, it is true that the recently launched protease inhibitors to treat HIV/AIDS are a remarkable breakthrough. They have opened up the possibility of AIDS becoming a chronic disease, which the patient lives with, rather than an inevitable death sentence. But you may not have heard the full story; the long-term effects of the drugs are unknown, they are unaffordable for the majority of AIDS patients, and treatment with them involves a complex dosing regime.

On the other hand, scare stories about the side effects of drugs are often taken out of context and, worse, people act upon the information they read. Remember those news reports, in 1995, about the increased risks of developing deep vein thrombosis with some brands of oral contraceptive. Thousands of women stopped taking their Pill immediately, terrified they would die of a stroke or heart attack. Many became pregnant as a result – thereby actually *doubling* their risk of a clot.

There is the same need for hard information and a balanced overview when it comes to discussing 'illegal' drugs and substance misuse. The arguments for and against the legalisation of cannabis, for instance, are often driven more by social, economic and political factors than by science.

In this book, I hope to give this broad and much-needed overview of the drugs we use – from medicines that save lives to drugs which enhance the quality of life. I have called it *Magic Molecules* because I have drawn quite heavily on the 'magic bullet' concept of Paul Ehrlich, the founding father of the modern pharmaceutical industry. Ehrlich's dream was to create safe and effective drugs which would home in upon their target in the body – be it an infectious bacterium or a cancer cell – with the precision of a 'magic bullet'.

Much of the discussion will be about pharmaceutical drugs. While I will celebrate some of the industry's remarkable breakthroughs – such as antibiotics, painkillers and hormonal contraceptives – I hope this book will also give readers cause to reflect on how well pharmaceutical drugs actually serve people's health needs.

In the West, heart disease and cancer are the leading causes of death and disability. So it is hardly surprising that many of the world's top selling drugs are for heart disease – it is a huge market. It is slightly harder to explain, in purely clinical terms, why the world's top selling drug is for ulcers – and not for cancer, or infection.

Worldwide, however, infectious disease remains the biggest killer, claiming the lives of 17 million people a year. We thought we had conquered infection with antibiotics – but these clinical weapons are fast losing their power as microbes evolve resistance to them, leaving us with a major public health problem. This has been caused, in part at least, by lack of vision, and reluctance to invest, on the part of the pharmaceutical industry.

And we still do not devote sufficient pharmaceutical resources to tropical diseases. Malaria kills three million people a year, one million of them children. But research into malaria receives only $60 million a year, compared to $140 million for asthma, $300 million for Alzheimer's disease and $950 million for AIDS. Is this fair?

But this book is not just about the pharmaceutical industry and its products. Drugs are molecules which have a biological effect. It really is not relevant whether the drug is legal or illegal, recreational or medicinal, synthetic or natural. The biology and chemistry of drugs crosses these boundaries. Therefore I have also looked at many of the drugs which are used for pleasure, and at the products of the health food industry; both are as important, in their way, as pharmaceutical drugs. In the end, this is a book about chemistry at its best – about how a 'magic molecule' finds a target within the body, and causes a biological response which may have a profound effect at many levels upon the individual.

Many drug names are mentioned in this book. Names whose first letters are lower case are generic names (the official medical names). Where appropriate I have also referred to UK brand names; these names begin with a capital letter.

Susan Aldridge

1

How drugs work

Glaring lights. Noise. Traffic congestion. Looming deadlines. None of it life-threatening, but enough to start up your body's favourite stress response – a tension headache. Muscles in your neck and scalp tighten, perhaps constricting nearby blood vessels. The affected tissue starts to produce chemicals called prostaglandins. These act on nearby nerve endings which, in turn, send messages to the brain producing the sensation of pain.

It may not be the best long-term solution (maybe you should give up that stressful job or take up yoga) but a couple of soluble aspirin tablets will kill that headache in about half an hour, by turning off prostaglandin production. The same goes for other everyday irritations such as toothache, menstrual cramps and rheumatic aches and pains.

Swallowing a dose of aspirin releases about two thousand million million million (2×10^{21}) pain-relieving molecules into the body. They won't all reach their target (the site of prostaglandin production), but experience of the drug over nearly 100 years has shown that this dose – around 600 milligrams – is enough to take care of most tension headaches.

The aspirin molecules first have to negotiate the digestive system to get into the bloodstream, which will carry them to the site of the pain (Fig. 1.1). The digestive system is basically a tube going from the mouth to the anus. It filters any molecules which enter it (food or drugs, that is) according to their size and chemical structure. Small, fat-soluble molecules pass easily though the walls of the small intestine into the bloodstream. Larger molecules such as proteins, fats and carbohydrates (the basic components of food) are chewed up into smaller fragments by the powerful acid juices of the stomach and the digestive enzymes produced by the stomach and pancreas. Other big molecules, like the cellulose in dietary fibre, pass unchanged through the gut.

Aspirin easily clears this first hurdle. It is a small molecule which is left alone by digestive enzymes and it is readily absorbed – mainly through the

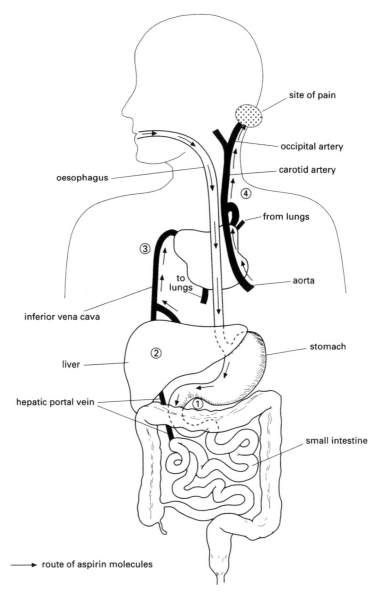

site of pain

occipital artery

carotid artery

oesophagus

④

from lungs

③

to lungs

aorta

inferior vena cava

② liver

stomach

hepatic portal vein

①

small intestine

⟶ route of aspirin molecules

Fig. 1.1. From pills to pain relief – the journey of an aspirin molecule. The route taken can be divided into four stages. (1) The pills dissolve in the stomach and nearly all the aspirin is absorbed by the stomach and small intestine. (2) Blood vessels from the stomach and small intestine carry the aspirin into the hepatic portal vein which leads to the liver. (3) From the liver, the hepatic vein takes the aspirin into the right atrium of the heart, which pumps blood

walls of the small intestine, although at least five per cent is absorbed through the stomach. Other drugs do not fare so well, as we shall see.

Next the aspirin molecules enter the liver, via the hepatic portal vein. The liver is a formidable obstacle for any drug; one of its main functions is to protect the body from 'foreign' molecules by dismantling them or modifying them in some other way (a process known as metabolism). Most drugs – and aspirin is no exception – are not found in the body under normal circumstances so the liver is bound to treat them with suspicion. The drug molecule that comes out of its first encounter with the liver (known in pharmacology jargon as the 'first pass') could be a very different animal from the one that went in.

The chemical name of aspirin is acetylsalicylic acid; put simply this means that its molecule consists of salicylic acid with a cluster of carbon, hydrogen and oxygen atoms known as an acetyl group tacked onto it (Fig. 1.2). The liver removes the acetyl group from at least some of the aspirin molecules, forming a compound called salicylic acid, itself a painkiller, and the historical precursor of aspirin.

Salicylic acid is an active ingredient of willow bark, and has been used as a folk remedy for pain and fever since the days of the great Greek physician Hippocrates (460–370 BC). By the 19th century it was widely used in the treatment of rheumatic fever, gout and arthritis. But salicylic acid is bitter and causes severe stomach irritation. So Felix Hoffman, a chemist at Bayer (the German company which had developed salicylic acid commercially) began to look for a related compound which would be a better drug, and came up with aspirin in 1899.

Some aspirin will sneak through the liver unchanged – the actual amount depending on the size of the dose, its formulation and the state of your liver. Along with the salicylic acid, it enters the general circulation and is transported around the body by the pumping action of the heart.

---

into the right ventricle, to the lungs for oxygenation, then back to the left atrium of the heart. (4) On the final leg of the journey, the aspirin passes from the left ventricle into the aorta and then to the carotid artery which serves the head and neck. The occipital artery is a branch of the carotid artery; it carries blood to the back of the head (the usual site of tension headache). It branches into smaller and smaller vessels, and through these aspirin eventually reaches the tissue where the prostaglandin pain signals are being produced.

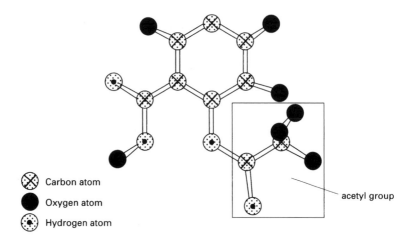

Fig. 1.2. The molecular structure of acetylsalicylic acid (aspirin). Each ball represents an atom, and each 'stick' a chemical bond joining two atoms together. Aspirin is formed when salicylic acid (the part of the molecule containing the ring) reacts with a compound containing the acetyl group.

Every part of the body now receives a dose of aspirin. But the aspirin molecules only have an effect in cells where prostaglandins are present. So they will cut off pain-producing prostaglandins and relieve that headache. But prostaglandins occur in the stomach too, where they help create a barrier of mucus which protects it from the acidic gastric juices. Aspirin turns off the production of these prostaglandins too. As a result, the stomach lining may become exposed to gastric juices, causing pain and possibly even the development of ulcers – especially if aspirin is being taken long-term.

Aspirin stops the production of prostaglandins for about four hours. The pain might come back, if the trigger that activates prostaglandins is still present. In this case, you may need another dose of aspirin; as the label on the packet says, repeat every four hours as necessary.

Once they have done their job the aspirin molecules (which are chemically changed into salicylic acid when they block prostaglandins, as we shall see) do not linger, but are swept away by the general circulation. They may pass through the liver again and be metabolised into smaller fragments, or they may pass straight out of the body via the kidneys. All the aspirin, in whatever form, has gone from the body within 24 hours.

This everyday story of pain relief illustrates the main problems in getting drugs to hit their targets. First it helps to know as precisely as possible what the target is. The way aspirin works was not known until nearly 70 years after its launch. In 1969 experiments carried out by John Vane and his team at the Royal College of Surgeons in London showed that the drug stops the synthesis of prostaglandins in damaged tissue (of which more in the next section).

Next, a way of delivering an effective dose of the drug into the body, to its target, and then out again has to be worked out. The information on a packet of aspirin-based painkillers contains a wealth of information on how the drug interacts with the body – digestive system, liver and kidneys. Look at any other drug, and the way it is delivered – tablets, injection or patch, for example – could be completely different, as could the daily dosage, the maximum safe dose and its formulation as a solid, soluble or slow release preparation.

Finally, it is important that the drug makes a reasonably 'clean' hit on the target. Side effects are the result of the drug hitting more than one target in the body. For instance, the action of aspirin on stomach prostaglandins produces bleeding and ulcers in some people.

Occasionally a new use for a drug can be developed from these side effects. For instance, prostaglandins in blood platelets generate a powerful clotting agent called thromboxane. Aspirin, in a lower dose than that used as a painkiller, stops the production of the prostaglandins that make thromboxane, and so can protect the cardiovascular system from the formation of dangerous blood clots that could trigger a heart attack or stroke. It is now routinely prescribed to people at risk; for instance, paramedics will give an aspirin to someone with a suspected heart attack as part of a first aid package, while people with angina or a history of heart attack can benefit from taking low-dose aspirin long-term (more on this in Chapter 5).

Many drugs work by homing in on molecular targets

There are hundreds of thousands of different molecules in the human body. Some are simple, like sodium chloride (common salt) and water; others like DNA, proteins and carbohydrates contain many thousands of atoms arranged to give a complex, three-dimensional structure. It is the interplay between these various molecules – biochemistry – which makes life possible. Digesting a meal, reading a newspaper, playing a game of badminton – these, and all other activities which involve muscular action, thought processes, or perception of the world around us are driven by biochemistry.

Biochemistry happens at the level of the cell – the basic building block of the body – although its results are often apparent at the level of the whole body. Two main groups of molecules, known as enzymes and receptors, lie at the heart of the biochemical activity of the cell. Most drugs work by interfering with the way in which either an enzyme or a receptor functions, with the knock-on effect of causing some change in the way the body functions.

Enzymes are biological catalysts. They speed up the chemical reactions that occur in the body so that they occur at a rate that is compatible with life. Without digestive enzymes, for example, it would take 50 years to break down the proteins, fats and carbohydrates in a typical meal into fragments that can be absorbed into the blood.

Crucial to an enzyme's action is its shape. Enzymes are proteins; they consist of a long chain of hundreds of basic building blocks called amino acids linked together. The chain is coiled up, under the influence of chemical bonds between the amino acids, into a roughly spherical shape. From a distance, all of the 50,000 to 100,000 enzymes in the human body would appear to have the same shape. Close up however, you would notice some subtle differences between them. Each enzyme has a cleft somewhere on its surface known as the active site. The chemical which the enzyme will transform into a product – known as the substrate – fits snugly into the active site like two pieces in a jigsaw (Fig. 1.3).

The enzyme's active site and the substrate have groups of atoms which attract one another, forming a weak chemical bond. Once the two have come together, the enzyme can get to work – perhaps snipping a chemical bond in the substrate, or creating a new one between two different substrates to make a larger molecule. Once the chemical action is over, the product molecule emerges from the enzyme, which is itself unchanged and ready to get to work on the next substrate molecule.

Each enzyme has its own specific substrate. For example pepsin, the enzyme that breaks down proteins, cannot stand in for amylase which breaks down starch. And if you put amylase and proteins together, nothing will happen.

If a drug molecule has a shape which is similar to that of a particular substrate, then it may drift into the active site – blocking the approach of the substrate. Such drugs are known as enzyme inhibitors (Fig. 1.3). Aspirin inhibits the enzyme cyclooxygenase (COX), which normally converts arachidonic acid (the substrate) into prostaglandins. The COX molecule is anchored to the membrane of a cell component called the endoplasmic reticulum. The arachidonic acid molecules are a component of this membrane,

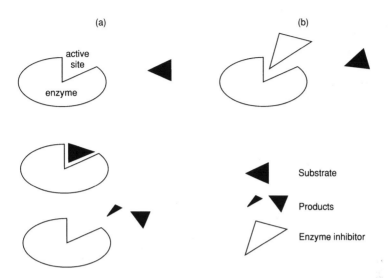

Fig. 1.3. Enzyme inhibitors. (a) The substrate approaches the active site of the enzyme, and binds to it – whereupon it is transformed into products. (b) An enzyme inhibitor binds to the active site in place of the substrate. Without binding to the active site, the substrate cannot be transformed into products. Note this figure is not to scale; substrates and inhibitors are normally much smaller than shown in comparison to the enzyme molecule.

and the active site is a long, narrow passage within the cyclooxygenase molecule. If an aspirin molecule gets into the passage, it blocks the entrance of arachidonic acid. So no prostaglandin is produced, and the net effect is to turn off the sensation of pain, as well as inhibiting the production of stomach mucus and thromboxane (Fig. 1.4). Drugs related to aspirin, such as ibuprofen and paracetamol, are thought to act in a similar way.

Many other drugs act as enzyme inhibitors, including angiotensin converting enzyme (ACE) inhibitors used in heart disease, certain antidepressants, penicillin (which acts on bacterial enzymes) and the new HIV protease inhibitors for the treatment of AIDS.

Like enzymes, receptors are proteins whose surfaces are pitted with nooks and crannies which smaller molecules can home in on. These 'keys' for the receptors' 'locks' are called ligands (Fig. 1.5). Receptors are found on the cell surface (whereas enzymes are usually inside the cell). They act as a link between the inside and outside of the cell.

Unlike an enzyme, a receptor does not transform the ligand which binds to it. Instead the act of binding sends a signal to the cell – causing it to

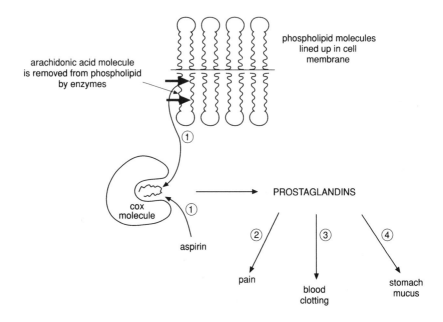

Fig. 1.4. Cyclooxygenase and the action of aspirin. The cell membrane bounding the interior of the cell is composed of a double layer of fatty molecules called phospholipids. Arachidonic acid, the substrate of cyclooxygenase (COX), is derived from a phospholipid molecule. It fits into the active site of COX (1) and enzymic action transforms it into a prostaglandin. But aspirin and related drugs also fit, to a greater or lesser extent, into the active site, blocking the enzymic action. Prostaglandins, depending upon where in the body they are produced, lead to pain (2), blood clotting via the action of thromboxane (3) or production of stomach mucus (4). Aspirin's action on COX can affect all three functions.

start up some biochemical activity which will culminate in a physiological response. So the ligand has an 'action at a distance' effect; it does not need to enter the cell to affect it. Hormones, and brain chemicals called neurotransmitters are two important classes of ligand. For instance, when the hormone insulin binds to its receptor it signals to the cells that there is plenty of glucose in the bloodstream. The cell responds by taking steps to store some of this in the liver, and other parts of the body, so that glucose levels in the bloodstream stay more or less constant.

So it is possible to manipulate the actions of cells by using drugs that bind to receptors. Some drugs – known as agonists – have a 'positive' effect, making the cell do what it does when its natural ligand binds. Morphine, a

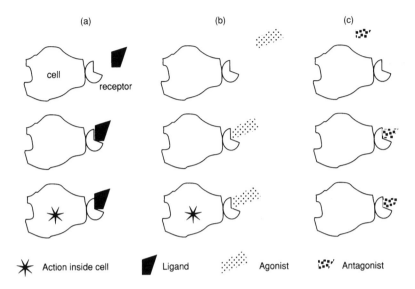

Fig. 1.5. Receptor agonists and antagonists. (a) A ligand approaches a cell surface receptor and binds to it. This sets off a cascade of biochemical reactions inside the cell which result in a physiological effect. (b) An agonist molecule acts similarly to the natural ligand, also producing action inside the cell. (c) An antagonist molecule merely binds to the cell surface receptor, blocking access to the ligand. It does not produce any action inside the cell.

drug used to relieve severe pain in cancer and heart attack patients, is an example of a receptor agonist. It binds to so-called opioid receptors in brain cells which normally respond to endorphins, the body's natural painkillers.

Other drugs bind to receptors but do not cause the cell to respond to them. They have a 'negative' effect and are known as receptor antagonists or blockers; when they are in position on the receptor, the ligand that normally binds to it is denied access, hence the blocking effect.

Important drugs in this category include the beta blockers, which are used to treat high blood pressure and heart disease. They act on so-called beta-adrenergic receptors which normally respond to the hormone adrenaline. This is the 'fight or flight' hormone which puts the body on 'red alert' by increasing blood pressure, heart rate, and breathing. Beta blockers counteract these effects; they decrease the heart rate and so lower blood pressure and reduce the workload on the heart.

There are many other ways in which drugs can act. Some interfere with the normal traffic of substances in and out of cells. The ion channel blockers are an important group in this category. Ion channels are tiny pores in the cell membrane that allow the passage of minerals such as calcium and sodium. When calcium ions pass through an ion channel, the end result is muscle contraction. Calcium antagonists, such as verapamil, can block the ion channel on heart muscle cells and so reduce the strength of the muscle contractions of the heart. Like the beta blockers, this has the effect of reducing the heart's workload, and so helps in cases of heart failure or angina.

There are also drugs which do not interfere directly with the body's chemistry, but remedy deficiencies in the supply levels of vitamins, minerals and enzymes. For instance, iron is needed to make the oxygen-carrying pigment haemoglobin. Iron deficiency can lead to anaemia, which is characterised by symptoms such as weakness, breathlessness and faintness. According to a report carried out by the British Nutrition Foundation up to ten per cent of women could be deficient in iron – either because of heavy periods, faulty diet, or both. If they are not able to boost their iron levels by eating more iron-rich foods such as meat or fortified cereals, they might be prescribed iron tablets, which contain ferrous sulphate, an easily absorbed form of the mineral.

Not all biochemical deficiencies are so easily remedied, and some can be life-threatening. Around one per cent of the population suffers from an inherited single-gene disorder. Genes are the blueprints from which enzymes and other proteins, such as haemoglobin, are synthesised. Defective genes may have a profound effect upon cellular biochemistry by giving wrong instructions for the synthesis of these proteins. In genetic disease, a key protein may be missing from the cell entirely, or it may be made in a form which does not work properly.

Some 5700 single-gene disorders have been discovered. Some are extremely rare and some are fatal before birth. Many are still poorly understood, usually because the gene affected is unknown. However, some single-gene disorders – such as haemophilia and cystic fibrosis – have been intensively studied. Therapy for these diseases consists of supplying the protein which the patient lacks. In the commonest form of haemophilia, for example, the missing or defective protein is known as factor VIII. Without factor VIII the blood cannot clot properly and the patient suffers from prolonged bleeding after dental treatment, for instance, or perhaps spontaneous internal bleeding into the joints with swelling and intense pain.

The development of drugs for haemophilia owes a great deal to advances in gene technology. The first treatment was with factor VIII extracted from human blood. This is effective, but puts the patient at risk of infection from blood-borne viruses such as hepatitis and HIV. Indeed thousands of haemophiliacs developed AIDS in the 1980s as a result of treatment with factor VIII. Genetic engineering techniques – of which more in Chapter 11 – have allowed the manufacture of factor VIII and many other therapeutic human proteins without the need to use human tissue.

Right dose, right place, right time

For each drug there is a minimum effective dose which will produce the required response in the body. What happens if a bigger dose is given depends on the drug, and the patient. For some drugs, such as the antibiotic gentamicin – which is used to treat eye infections as well as life-threatening septicaemia – toxic effects kick in fairly quickly after the minimum effective dose. Such drugs are said to have a small therapeutic index. To find the therapeutic index, you divide the minimum dose which gives toxic effects by the minimum effective dose. The therapeutic index of gentamicin is 3; if three times the minimum effective dose was accidentally prescribed, then the effect on the patient could be disastrous. In contrast another antibiotic, benzylpenicillin, has a therapeutic index of over 100. So if a patient does not seem to be responding to the minimum effective dose, a doctor can push the dose up without worrying too much about toxicity. Everyone responds differently to the drugs they are prescribed; drugs with a high therapeutic index allow these individual responses to be accommodated more easily.

The minimum effective dose is the one which will allow enough drug molecules to reach their target, whether they are given as a pill, injection or in some other form. The method of delivery is crucial, and depends on how the body handles the drug.

Pills are the most popular form of medicine; they are convenient, painless and easy to take. But, as discussed earlier, some drugs have difficulty in getting from the mouth into the bloodstream because of the way the gut and liver handle them. Largish molecules such as the antibiotic cefotaxime, which is used in the treatment of meningitis, cannot easily penetrate the walls of the small intestine. Typically less than 20 per cent of a dose of cefotaxime, and related antibiotics, ends up in the circulation. Other drugs such as the anti-depressants imipramine and doxepin run into trouble when they get to the liver, which breaks down more than half of the molecules in the given dose. A drug's ability to negotiate the gut and liver is known as its bioavailability. If all the dose gets through, the bioavailability has a value of 1; if none does, the bioavailability is zero. With drugs that have a low bioavailability there are two options – either adjust the dose accordingly, or deliver the drug by some means other than a pill.

An estimated 420,000 people in Britain, and around 10 million world-wide, take insulin every day to control their diabetes (for more on insulin and diabetes see Chapter 4). Insulin is a peptide drug. Like a protein, a peptide consists of many chemically linked amino acid units. But peptides contain fewer than 100 amino acids, while proteins contain more than 100. The enzyme pepsin in the stomach breaks the links between the amino acids of both peptides and proteins. So the bioavailability of insulin is zero. Until recently, injections have been the only way diabetics could get insulin into their bodies.

An intravenous injection is the most rapid way of getting a drug into the circulation. However only medically trained people should give intravenous injections, because you need to be able to find a vein, and be sure not to inject an air bubble from the syringe into the circulation. If this finds its way to the heart it could form a dangerous airlock obstructing the outflow of blood to the lungs – causing breathlessness, chest pain and maybe even heart failure.

Injections are sometimes given into the muscle of the buttocks, shoulder or thigh; this is the way nurses usually give injections – of painkillers or vaccines, for example. Muscle has a rich blood supply so the drug quickly finds its way into the circulation. Diabetics usually give themselves subcut-aneous injections – under the skin of the upper arm, thigh or abdomen. Since twice-daily injections (a common regime for controlling blood sugar in diabetes) are painful and inconvenient, insulin has become the proving ground for some exciting new drug delivery technologies.

Instead of the traditional syringe and needles, many diabetics use a pen injector fitted with a cartridge of insulin. They use a dial to measure out the dose, and a plunger to inject it. Another option is a jet injector in which a stream of high pressure air pushes insulin through the skin without a needle. These are expensive, and some patients still find them as painful as conven-tional injections. Scientists in Oxford are trying to improve on this design with a supersonic injector, in which a pellet of compressed helium bursts when the syringe is depressed. The gas, travelling at twice the speed of sound, carries the powdered drug through the skin. All you feel is a light touch. The device should be available a year or so after it has been fully tested. A similar device which uses compressed carbon dioxide as a propel-lant has already been used to deliver injections of hepatitis B vaccine to 60,000 or so schoolchildren in New York.

Drugs can be delivered directly through the skin via patches. However, the skin does present a formidable barrier to the entry of 'foreign' substances, and the patch method is usually only suitable for the delivery of low doses. Scopolamine – a drug for travel sickness – hormone replacement therapy and nicotine can all be given by skin patches. Research into skin patches for painkillers, high blood pressure medication and anti-depressants is well underway.

However, for insulin delivery through the skin there is is a need to enhance penetration. One method that might achieve this is iontophoresis, which uses 'active patches' to drive drugs painlessly through sweat glands or hair follicles, under the influence of a tiny electric current supplied from a miniature battery. All the patient feels is a tingling sensation. However, so far the technique has met with only limited success in the delivery of insulin.

Diabetics can also get around the chore of daily injections by using devices that pump insulin into the body. These fit into the abdomen and deliver insulin through a tube into the peritoneal space (between the abdominal wall and the organs of the abdominal cavity). To ensure that the pump delivers the right amount of insulin patients have to monitor their blood sugar three or four times a day and adjust the dose accordingly. In the future, the pumps could be fitted with advanced programming and memory software. Results from recent trials of implantable pumps show they give better blood sugar control than injections, and improved quality of life. The most sophisticated pump technology, currently under trial in animals, is the closed loop system in which a glucose monitoring device is automatically linked to the pump. Blood sugar readings are automatically translated into the amount of insulin required by the body.

Drugs like insulin can also enter the body through the mucous membranes – the wet surfaces – instead of through the skin. So far, however, trials of the nasal spray on patients have been disappointing – nasal insulin does not control blood sugar nearly as well as injections. Insulin eye drops seem to work better, at least in animals. The eye drops are actually absorbed into the circulation via the nasal mucosa, which they reach through blood vessels in the face. They raise the level of insulin in the blood and this, in turn, has been shown to control blood sugar. The eye drops probably work better than the nasal spray because it is just easier to deliver a consistent volume of the drug into the eye than to the nose.

There is currently great interest in giving insulin, and many other drugs, by inhalation. The lungs have a high absorptive area and their tissue walls are thinner than blood capillaries – which speeds up absorption. Inhaled drugs are given as a dry powder (the particles must be less than 5 µm in diameter to be effective) or as a nebuliser, which is a mist of fine droplets containing the drug.

In in the next year or so there may even be insulin pills on offer. The trick to smuggling drugs past the stomach, which would otherwise attack them, is to encase them in some kind of inert compartment. Liposomes – fatty capsules which surround a dose of a drug – have been tried as a container for insulin, but with little success. But a container made of a synthetic polymer is showing more promise.

Timing of insulin injections to meet the body's needs is vital. There is no set regime, but many diabetics inject three times a day before meals, and once again at bedtime – trying to mimic the body's natural ebb and flow of insulin production. It is now becoming apparent that the timing of other drugs may have an important impact on their effectiveness by tuning in with the body's physiological rhythms. For instance, the acidity of urine is greater at night than during the day. Alkaline drugs – which react with acids – are most easily removed in nocturnal urine. They therefore stay in the body for longer if they are administered during the day rather than at bedtime. With acidic drugs, the reverse is true.

The symptoms of some illnesses are known to vary on a 24-hour cycle and medication can be given on a schedule that takes account of this. For example, 80 per cent of asthma attacks occur in the middle of the night. Bronchodilator drugs which relieve asthma have their greatest effect on the lungs if given early in the morning or late in the day, and the least effect around noon. It has been shown that the best control of asthma comes from taking drugs morning and evening, rather than giving doses equally spaced throughout the day.

A daily rhythm is also seen arthritis. The pain of rheumatoid arthritis is worst in the morning, while that of osteoarthritis peaks in the later afternoon. So for maximum relief of rheumatoid arthritis, aspirin should be given in the late evening, while for osteoarthritis it should be given in mid-afternoon. Another factor to be taken into account, however, is that gastric irritation from aspirin is greater in the morning than in the evening.

Drugs which are toxic to the kidney, such as the anti-cancer drug cisplatin, are best given in the late afternoon when the kidneys are most active (and can more effectively remove the drug), while administration late at night does most damage, because this is when the kidneys are at their least active. Minimising toxic effects by careful timing means bigger doses can be given, increasing the overall benefit to the patient.

That this approach – known as chronotherapy – works was shown by William Hrushesky and his team at the University of Minnesota Hospital in the mid-1980s. They took two small groups of women with advanced ovarian cancer and treated them with two anti-cancer drugs, adriamycin and cisplatin. The only difference between the groups was in the timing of the drug doses. One group took adriamycin in the morning and cisplatin in the evening. In the other group, the timings were reversed. The first group experienced far fewer side effects – so their doctors were able to give them more of the drug, maximising their chances of beating the tumour.

In another trial, chemotherapy for childhood leukaemia was given either in the morning or in the afternoon. The latter group, followed up several years later, had a two and a half times greater cure rate than the former. Timing of anti-cancer drugs is not just important from the point of view of side effects. Since many of them rely on killing rapidly-dividing cancer cells (see also Chapter 7), they are more likely to be effective if they are given at a time of day when normal cells are not dividing, so that they can more cleanly target the cancer cells (which do not have a daily rhythm – they divide all the time).

To date, chronotherapy has not made a great impact upon how drugs are prescribed. But one day the label on a bottle of pills may say 'take at 9 am, 3 pm and 7 pm' instead of 'take three times a day before meals'.

Hitting the wrong targets: the problem of side effects

The most important factor in making a drug effective is the one that is most often overlooked by doctors. The patient has to actually take the drug for it to work. Research shows that up to half of patients with serious chronic illness do not take their tablets as prescribed. Some do not even collect their prescription from the chemist, others stop taking their pills after a few days. And many do not admit non-compliance to their doctors for fear of upsetting them.

A famous non-complier was the world's first heart transplant patient, Louis Washkansky. In a recent TV interview, his widow revealed that Washkansky had refused to take prescribed medication for the heart failure that led him to the brink of death. We can only speculate – but supposing he had taken the pills? Maybe there would have been less need for the operation. And perhaps he would have survived for longer than 18 days after receiving his new heart.

A recent survey suggests that non-compliance among transplant patients often continues after surgery, when they must start on a life-long programme of drugs to stop rejection of the new organ. One in five patients receiving a new kidney stops taking anti-rejection drugs. Most die or suffer organ rejection as a result. The latter group has to go back on dialysis, or await a second transplant (both options push another kidney patient back in the queue for treatment). The main reason for this surprising non-compliance is that many transplant patients think of the operation as a total cure, and cannot come to terms with taking up to 20 pills a day to keep themselves well. Like many people they just 'don't like taking pills'.

People on medication for high blood pressure, asthma, depression, schizophrenia, and epilepsy also have a strong tendency to reject their drugs. Some of the reasons are rooted in human psychology; patients fear addiction, are absent-minded, or fail to appreciate the seriousness of their condition.

Calendar packs, depot injections and slow-release formulations may make medication easier to take. And better communication between doctor and patient can improve compliance. This can range from simply giving information and reassurance to active supervision of the patient, ensuring that they do take the drug as prescribed. The last option might sound a bit authoritarian, but in some circumstances it really does work. Directly observed therapy (DOT) as it is known was adopted in New York City and in other parts of the United States to improve the poor compliance rate among TB patients. Many were homeless, jobless and living generally disorganised lives – hardly surprising then that they found it hard to stick to a six-month treatment schedule involving a cocktail of antibiotic drugs. In DOT, nurses watch the patients taking their pills every day – either in the clinic, at the patient's home, or at his place of work. In Tarrant County, Texas, DOT cut the relapse rate in a group of TB patients from 20 per cent to five per cent – and at a time when TB rates elsewhere were on the increase. Far from resenting the interference in their lives, patients appreciated DOT, because of the bond that developed between them and the nurses. Word spread, and new patients have begun asking for DOT when they check into the clinic with TB.

But even the best-motivated people may have to stop a potentially useful drug because they are suffering from unacceptable side effects (defined as adverse signs and symptoms appearing alongside the therapeutic effects of a drug). The human body is so complex that no drug is completely 'clean' in its actions. The drug is bound to encounter molecules which resemble its target. Whether it hits these too – causing side effects – depends upon just how specific it is to the target. Better understanding of the molecular structure of targets (more about this in Chapter 2) allows fine-tuning of the structure of drug molecules; these can be turned into medication with fewer side effects.

For example aspirin and related drugs inhibit the cyclooxygenase (COX) enzyme, both in the stomach and in any painful, inflamed area of the body, and thereby turn off the production of prostaglandins. But stomach prostaglandins – as mentioned earlier – play a vital role, producing mucus that protects the stomach lining. Without them irritation, bleeding and ulceration may occur. If only aspirin could distinguish between COX in the stomach and COX in the painful area, and just hit on the latter and spare the stomach. This wish is now becoming a reality as a new generation of 'super-aspirins' makes its way onto the market. In 1991 Japanese scientists showed that COX in the stomach and COX in painful, inflamed tissue were actually slightly different enzymes – now known as COX 1 and COX 2 respectively. The search was on for molecules that hit COX 2 but not COX 1. The first 'super-aspirin', meloxicam, has twice the affinity for COX 2 as for COX 1 and has been shown to cause significantly fewer side effects. It has recently been launched in Europe, Latin America and South Africa to relieve the pain and inflammation of arthritis. And things could get even better – many 'super-aspirins' under development have a 200-fold greater affinity for COX2 than COX 1.

There is a similar effort underway to find better drugs for schizophrenia that target the receptors thought to be involved in the illness, without hitting other similar receptors in the brain that are involved in control of movement. Existing drugs home in on both types – leaving the patient with an array of unpleasant side effects (for more on this see Chapter 8).

Medicines most associated with side effects include antibiotics, anticoagulants, tranquillisers and non-steroidal anti-inflammatory agents (used as painkillers and for rheumatic conditions such as arthritis). It is estimated that 0.3 per cent of hospital admissions are because of drug side effects and five per cent of patients suffer from side effects on medication (the real figure could, of course, be much higher than this; not all patients report side effects to their doctor, and not all doctors pass the information on to colleagues, a medical journal, or the manufacturer). The commonest side effects are nausea and diarrhoea, drowsiness, dizziness, and skin rashes. A recent survey of 250 British GPs (family doctors) showed that between 10 and 20 per cent of patients prescribed non-steroidal anti-inflammatory drugs, such as ibuprofen, for arthritis and similar conditions stopped taking them because of side effects, of which by far the most frequent was stomach irritation.

Many side effects are predictable from the way the drug acts – even without the detailed molecular knowledge described earlier that has led to the development of new types of aspirin-like drugs. Diuretic drugs, which relieve heart failure and are used to treat hypertension, do so by reducing the amount of fluid in the body. This means patients could complain of more frequent urination which may disturb their sleep. It is also possible that they could lose the mineral potassium in the fluid leaving the body.

And it is not just therapeutic drugs which give rise to side effects. Caffeine in strong coffee can cause palpitations, cocaine causes weight loss and exhaustion, and amphetamines can lead to paranoia, lethargy and depression.

Occasionally side effects are positive. The anti-hypertensive drug minoxidil causes increased hair growth in some people. Rubbing a solution of minoxidil onto the scalp has now been turned into an effective cure for baldness; 85 per cent of people trying it said hair loss stopped, and 37 per cent found that new hair began to grow.

Some side effects have more to do with the patient as an individual than they do with the chemistry of the drug molecule. Usually these reactions are allergies, similar to the allergies some people have to peanuts or cow's milk. Common drugs which induce allergic reactions include aspirin and penicillin. The symptoms of allergic reactions include skin rashes and swelling. More rarely a life-threatening condition known as anaphylactic shock can develop – sometimes within minutes – once penicillin molecules, say, are introduced into the body.

What happens is that the immune system perceives the 'foreign' penicillin molecule as an 'enemy' and mobilises for attack. This involves the release of irritating chemicals such as histamine from cells of the immune system, called mast cells. The chemicals cause a number of physiological effects such as increased blood flow and swelling which serve the body well in moderation, and under the influence of a genuine threat such as an invading microbe. But in the case of anaphylactic shock the response goes into overdrive and produces dangerous swelling of the throat, which makes the victim gasp for breath, collapse of the circulation, heart failure – and, unless prompt action is taken, death. One to ten per cent of the population is allergic to penicillin (people who have other allergies appear to be particularly at risk).

A smaller number – perhaps one in 5000 – actually go into anaphylactic shock, and the condition causes around one death a year in the UK.

Many people – especially the very sick and the elderly – take more than one drug at a time. Sometimes this can be beneficial – a case of the whole being greater than the sum of its parts – as, for example, when a cocktail of antibiotics is prescribed for a serious infectious disease such as TB. Bacteria which are resistant to the effects of one of the drugs (see also Chapter 4) will then, hopefully, be knocked out by one of the others.

More often, though, drugs interact to give an adverse effect. Nearly half of hospital patients take six or more drugs. The number of possible interactions between the drugs increases steeply with the number of drugs prescribed. If someone is on two drugs there can only be one interaction between them. If they are taking seven, then there are 21 possible interactions.

Minimising drug–drug interactions is where the skill of the prescriber is really tested. For example, they will know that a drug with a narrow therapeutic index – like the heart drug digoxin – is more sensitive to any second drug that enhances its effect. The interaction tends to tip the digoxin over into its toxic range. The patient may well start to suffer side effects when a second – or subsequent – drug is added to their programme. Removing, replacing or reducing the dose of the interacting drug may well eliminate the side effects.

A good understanding of how each drug acts in the body means that most drug interactions are predictable – although there is always the odd surprise. So, if two drugs have similar effects, their effects will be additive. Aspirin and warfarin both thin the blood – even if the aspirin is being taken for pain or inflammation relief – and together might lead to unwanted bleeding, say in the stomach. Alcohol has a depressant effect on the central nervous system (CNS). It may produce drowsiness, unconsciousness and even coma when taken with other CNS depressants such as tranquillisers. Other drugs have opposite effects and may act to cancel each other so the patient gets no benefit from either. Steroids cause water and salt retention which tends to raise the blood pressure. Taken with a patient's regular anti-hypertensive medication, they may tend to cancel its effects.

Other drugs just interfere with one another. For instance, a woman may get pregnant if she takes antibiotics alongside oral contraceptives. Antibiotics may reduce the number of bacteria in the gut, as well as wiping out those responsible for any infection. But these gut bacteria are responsible for activating the hormones in the contraceptive – knocking them out may make the Pill lose its effectiveness.

An individual response

You can never be quite sure how someone will respond to a prescribed drug, because people are more than just a collection of enzymes, receptors and cells. Age, sex, weight, condition of health, and genetics all play a part in how a drug acts in a given individual.

The state of someone's liver and kidneys is particularly important because this determines how well they will handle the breakdown and elimination of a medicine. For example, by age 65 kidney function is down to three-quarters of the efficiency of the kidneys of a 25-year-old, so drugs tend to linger in the body. Older people therefore need smaller doses of most drugs. Babies and young children have immature kidneys and livers, so need smaller doses of drugs than adults, because their bodies are less able to break them down (check on any patient information and you will note that many drugs are not recommended at all for the under-12s).

There are also genetic differences in the way people respond to drugs. Nearly ten per cent of Europeans have an impaired ability to break down some drugs. This means that the drugs will be more powerful than expected, because they linger in the circulation. For instance, some drugs for hypertension lower the blood pressure below normal levels in these people. Other people may have a greater than normal ability to break drugs down – they may not respond so well to a normally effective dose (more about tailoring drugs to the individual in Chapter 11).

Pregnant women form a special category when it comes to taking drugs of any kind, because the drug can pass through the placenta to the developing foetus. Surprisingly, perhaps, little account was taken of the effect of drugs on the unborn child until the thalidomide tragedy came to light in the 1960s. Thalidomide, which came onto the market in 1956, was prescribed for a wide range of conditions from influenza to insomnia. It was even sold without prescription. Then, in 1961, clinics in West Germany reported nearly 500 cases of a rare congenital deformity in which the limbs are shortened or non-existent. Puzzled, doctors blamed X-rays, contraceptives and hormones – until surveys of mothers with affected babies showed that the majority had taken thalidomide during pregnancy. Perhaps 20 per cent of women who had taken the drug in the crucial period – between 37 and 54 days into the pregnancy – gave birth to an affected child. The world-wide toll of thalidomide survivors was to reach 10,000. In West Germany, only 5000 out of 10,000 affected survived. Thalidomide was rapidly with-drawn from the market, in 1961, although it is now used again, in a limited way, in the treatment of leprosy – for which it is an effective drug.

Shortly after the thalidomide scandal came news that girls whose mothers had been taking diethylstilboestrol (DES) during pregnancy were turning up with rare vaginal and cervical cancers. DES is a hormone which was taken by literally millions of women in the US and in Europe between 1948 and 1971 to prevent miscarriage. The drug was withdrawn in the 1970s when it became apparent that it damaged the developing reproductive system of the foetus. Besides the cancers, 40 per cent of exposed girls had deformities of their reproductive organs. And as they reached childbearing age themselves, many experienced recurrent miscarriage and a higher than normal rate of ectopic pregnancies. Nor were exposed boys unscathed – they show lower sperm counts and abnormal testicular development.

With hindsight the DES disaster was predictable. Hormones act as chemical signals during foetal development. Being exposed to the wrong signals at the wrong time can disrupt the normal developmental pathway giving rise to a wide range of deformities. More recent studies have linked hor-mone-like chemicals in the environment with sexual developmental abnor-malities in many species of wildlife including whales, alligators, fish and sea-gulls. The same chemicals have been linked, tentatively, with decreasing sperm counts and increasing rates of breast, prostate and testicular cancer.

Badly burned by thalidomide and DES, both doctors and prospective parents began to show a great deal more concern over drugs that were taken in pregnancy. The thalidomide tragedy itself led to profound changes in the way medicines were controlled in the UK. In May 1963, Kenneth Robinson, the Health Minister, said: 'The House and the public suddenly woke up to the fact that any drug manufacturer could market any product, however inadequately tested, however dangerous, without having to satisfy any inde-pendent body as to its efficacy and safety and the public was almost uniquely unprotected in this respect.' The UK's Medicines Act (1968) now sets a formal legal framework within which pharmaceutical drugs are evaluated.

Unfortunately, there is little hard information about how most drugs affect the foetus because pharmaceutical companies are understandably reluctant to carry out trials on pregnant women. What we do know comes from experience with various drugs in pregnant women over a period of time.

Some authorities such as the United States Food and Drug Administration (FDA) have created classes of drug based on their teratogenicity – or potential for causing developmental abnormality in a foetus. While no drug can be said to be completely without risk, those in class A – including paracetamol and penicillin – are thought to be relatively harm-free. Classes B, C and D carry an increasing risk of teratogenicity, while those in class X are not to be used in pregnancy at all.

An example of a class X drug is isotretinoin, which is used in the treatment of very severe acne. It is taken by mouth, and is meant to be a drug of last resort when both treatments applied to the skin and antibiotic tablets have failed. Isotretinoin can cause profound physical and mental handicap in an exposed foetus. In 1988, the FDA brought in a series of preventative measures to protect unborn children from isotretinoin. Women have to show evidence of a negative pregnancy test, for example, before the drug can be prescribed. A survey showed that almost all women knew of the dangers of isotretinoin in pregnancy, thanks to the new restrictions, although a substantial minority – around a third – had not been required to show evidence of a negative pregnancy test.

The foetus is particularly vulnerable during the first three months of pregnancy, and women are often advised to avoid all drugs during this time – even some over the counter medicines such as vitamins (high doses of vitamin A, in particular, could cause profound physical and mental defects). But sometimes it is riskier for a woman not to take drugs – if she had epilepsy, or diabetes, for example. An epileptic fit might cause more damage to a developing foetus than an anti-epileptic drug.

The damage a drug may do to the unborn child depends upon its type of action. Anti-cancer drugs, for instance, stop cells dividing and their main effect on the foetus occurs in the first 16 days of pregnancy when it is still just a ball of cells. Others cause damage later on, from 17 to 60 days, when the organs are being formed. For example, the group of drugs called the ACE inhibitors which are used to treat heart disease and high blood pressure halt the development of the kidneys.

Many women might take drugs without knowing they are pregnant. By the time they do become aware of their condition – often about six weeks into the pregnancy – the central nervous system, ears and eyes of the baby will already have been formed. So ideally all sexually active women of child-bearing age should be prescribed drugs of low teratogenic potential – paracetamol, for example.

2

From penicillin to Prozac: introducing pharmaceutical drugs

In the UK today there are around 6000 different drugs, available either on prescription or over the counter. They range from antibiotics, anaesthetics and painkillers, to drugs that treat heart disease, cancer, ulcers, and depression.

The pharmaceutical industry has grown tremendously over the last 50 years or so; in 1934 doctors had only a thousand medicines to offer their patients. Aspirin was one of the first drugs to be manufactured, by the German company Bayer in 1899. But the industry did not really take off until the 1930s with the development of the antibiotic Prontosil, which was soon followed by the launch of penicillin and related drugs.

In the 1940s and 1950s drugs to treat conditions such as epilepsy, allergy and mental illness were discovered. Research and development continued to gather pace – and between 1970 and 1990, over 400 new drugs were introduced in the UK alone.

Drugs are big business: the pharmaceutical industry is said to be worth $256 billion per annum, and to be growing at around ten per cent a year. In the UK, for instance, pharmaceuticals had a trade surplus of £2133 million in 1995, second only to North Sea oil.

The top 20 worldwide best-sellers (Table 1) are mostly treatments for infection, heart disease and digestive system disorders such as ulcers. Of the 484 new drugs coming onto the UK market in the period from 1972–1995, the top three categories were diseases of the central nervous system (77 drugs), infection (76 drugs) and cardiovascular disease (73 drugs). But there are still many conditions, as we shall see, for which there are few or no pharmaceutical drugs.

Discovering and developing new pharmaceuticals is a costly business. On average it takes 12 years to bring a drug onto the market from its initial discovery, and the total bill comes to over $350 million. Over this period of

Table 1. *The world's top-selling drugs*[a]

Name[b]	Used to treat	Source[c]	Sales[d]
Zantac (ranitidine)	Ulcers, indigestion	Synthetic	3.78
Renitec (enalapril)	High blood pressure, heart failure	Natural	2.31
Losec (omeprazole)	Ulcers	Synthetic	2.30
Prozac (fluoxetine)	Depression	Synthetic	2.07
Zocor (simvastatin)	High cholesterol	Natural	1.96
Capoten (captopril)	High blood pressure, heart failure	Natural	1.54
Zovirax (acyclovir)	Viral infections	Synthetic	1.45
Ciproxin (ciprofloxacin)	Bacterial infections	Synthetic	1.43
Voltaren (diclofenac)	Arthritis	Synthetic	1.32
Augmentin (amoxycillin and clavulanic acid)	Bacterial infections	Natural[e]	1.30
Sandimmun (cyclosporin)	Supresses immunity after organ transplantation	Natural	1.29
Adalat (nifedipine)	High blood pressure, angina	Synthetic	1.27
Mevacor (lovastatin)	High cholesterol	Natural	1.25
Istin (amlodipine)	High blood pressure, angina	Synthetic	1.24
Procardia (nifedipine)	High blood pressure, angina	Synthetic	1.14
Mevalotin (pravastatin)	High cholesterol	Natural	1.12
Cardizem (diltiazem)	High blood pressure, angina	Synthetic	1.10
Rocepin (cefatriaxone)	Bacterial infections	Natural	1.09
Klacid (clarithromycin)	Bacterial infections	Natural	1.05
Tylenol (paracetamol)	Pain	Synthetic	1.05

[a]Worldwide figures for 1995 (source *Scrip* magazine)
[b]Brand name given with generic name in brackets
[c]Natural products include those that come indirectly from natural materials. Cyclosporin and Mevacor are completely natural, being extracted from fungi
[d]Figures are in billions of dollars
[e]The clavulanic acid component is synthetic

time, it will pass through various stages (Fig. 2.1). In the first stage, basic research, hundreds – or even thousands – of chemical compounds are evaluated to identify one or more 'lead' compounds which are worthy of extra attention.

The most promising lead passes through to the second stage, pre-clinical development, and becomes known as a candidate drug. In pre-clinical development a candidate drug is groomed for stardom by a multidisciplinary team. Chemists investigate various synthetic routes to the candidate drug, and may also synthesise related compounds. They also look at whether it will be practical and cost-effective to scale up production from the gram quantities which suffice for laboratory research to the kilograms required to make tablets or injections to satisfy an international market. Pharmacologists look at how the body might handle the drug, addressing questions such as toxicity, lifetime, and efficacy – first using biological molecules and cells in test-tube studies, then graduating to experiments on animals. This will lead to decisions about how best to deliver the new drug to get it to its target and keep it in the body for the required length of time.

A candidate drug that gets this far will pass to the third and final stage – clinical trials. This is where the drug is tested in humans, and news of its performance starts to trickle through to the general public via the media. If all goes well, the drug will then be launched onto the market. The failure rate in drug development is, however, enormous. Typically only one in 5000 compounds evaluated in the initial stages actually makes it into the pharmacy.

New technologies, such as computer modelling as an aid to drug discovery, and increased demands from the regulatory agencies, have pushed research and development costs up to 20 per cent of sales, compared to only four per cent in 1966. As soon as the decision to go for the development of a new drug is made (at the point where a lead compound is promoted to the status of candidate drug, that is), the company applies for a patent. This gives it exclusive rights to the drug's development and promotion for a period of 20 years – and a chance to recoup the money invested in it.

By the time the drug has reached the market place, there may only be a few years left on the patent (although it can now be extended under certain circumstances). Once the patent has expired, other companies are free to make cheap copies – known as generic drugs. As pressure on healthcare costs mounts, doctors are tending to prescribe generic drugs rather than brand names. There are no generic versions of Zantac yet (the UK patent on the first form of this, the world's best-selling drug has recently expired

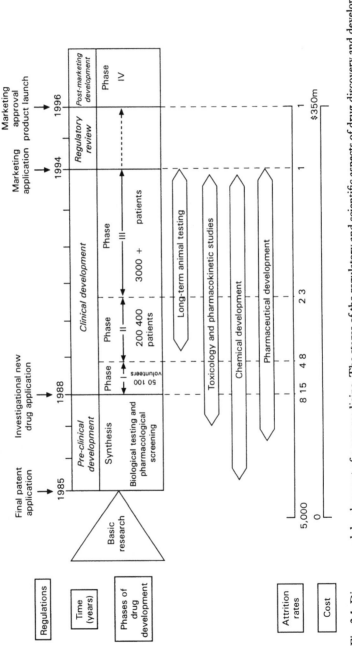

Fig. 2.1. Discovery and development of a new medicine. The stages of the regulatory and scientific aspects of drug discovery and development are displayed horizontally, along with the attrition or failure rates at each stage, and the cumulative cost. Source: Centre for Medicines Research, reproduced with permission.

however), but there are now dozens of medicines containing paracetamol, which first came onto the market in 1953.

A company might try to prolong the commercial lifetime of its drug by making it available without a prescription, selling direct to the consumer. Zantac, for example, is now available as an over-the-counter remedy for indigestion. General sale medicines such as aspirin, paracetamol and milk of magnesia are on sale in supermarkets and can be bought without supervision. The consumer is free to choose either the branded name or the generic copy, if there is one.

Most drugs are carbon-based and mimic body chemicals

If we picture an organism as infected by a certain species of bacterium, it will obviously be easy to effect a cure if substances have been discovered which have an exclusive affinity for these bacteria and act . . . on these alone while . . . they possess no affinity whatever for the normal constituents of the body, and cannot . . . have the least harmful, or other, effect on that body. Such substances would then be able to exert their full action exclusively on the parasite harboured within the organism, and would represent, . . . magic bullets which seek their target of their own accord.

The words of the German medical scientist Paul Ehrlich (1854–1915), spoken around 1905, first formulated the concept of a drug molecule as a magic bullet, homing in on its target and leaving the rest of the body unharmed. No one has ever found a magic bullet; all drugs have side effects and none achieves a desired action in all patients at all times. Yet the concept still drives drug discovery, and it is possible that advances in molecular biology, and better chemical technologies, may help us edge closer to Ehrlich's ideal.

Most drugs today are small, organic compounds. Organic chemistry is the chemistry of carbon, the element upon which life is based. Carbon is unique among the 92 naturally occurring elements in its ability to generate diversity when it bonds to other elements – principally hydrogen, oxygen, sulphur, phosphorus and chlorine. Carbon-based compounds range from small and simple, like methane (the main constituent of natural gas) which consists of just four hydrogen atoms bonded to one carbon, to huge and complex like the proteins, which may typically contain thousands of carbon atoms. Some organic compounds – like proteins and DNA – contain long strings of carbon atoms, while others, such as aspirin (Fig. 1.2), morphine and penicillin, contain rings of carbon atoms, sometimes interspersed with other atoms.

We saw in Chapter 1 that many drugs resemble the body's natural compounds – enzyme inhibitors and receptor agonists and antagonists, for example. So it is hardly surprising that drug molecules tend to be organic compounds. Most are small molecules, consisting of up to 50 atoms, mainly because traditionally these have been easiest for chemists to either make in the laboratory, or identify from natural sources such as plants.

But developments in molecular biology since the discovery of the structure of DNA in 1953 have led to an increasing emphasis on larger gene-based molecules. There has also been increasing interest in using proteins themselves as drugs (the impact of biotechnology on the pharmaceutical industry is discussed fully in Chapter 11).

Half the world's drugs come from nature . . .

In the past, all medicines came from plants and other natural sources. As modern chemistry developed, extraction and analysis of the active ingredients began to take over from the use of traditional medicines (although these still form the basis of herbal medicines around the world, as we shall see in Chapter 10). The first successful product of the 'grind and find' approach was the heart drug digitalis, which was derived from the foxglove by the Birmingham physician William Withering in 1796.

Today just over 50 per cent of all drugs in clinical use come, in some way, from natural products. Around half of these come from plants traditionally used in healing. Digitalis is still extracted from foxgloves and morphine still comes from poppies, but few other drugs are extracted directly from their original source these days. Among the 20 best-sellers only two fall into this category (see Table 1).

Sometimes a plant extract, or a microbial fermentation, will provide the raw material for the synthesis of a drug. For example, the cholesterol-lowering drug Zocor is a synthetic product derived from a fermentation extract of a fungus called *Aspergillus terreus*. Other drugs, like the anti-malarial quinine, are synthetic copies of a natural product. Many chemists view natural products as a treasure chest of novel molecules which they can elaborate in the laboratory. Khellin, a compound found in the fruit of a plant called *Ammi visnaga*, was the basis for the development of an anti-asthma drug, cromoglycate, and a heart drug, amiodarone.

There is huge untapped pharmaceutical potential in the natural world. Humans rely on the products of their brainpower – guns, tanks and money – to defend their interests. Plants, insects and microbes use chemical warfare. They manufacture their own weapons, known as secondary metabolites, and these are the compounds we exploit as drugs. Many fungi manufacture antibiotics, chemicals which kill competing microbes, while snake venoms contain a mixture of compounds with important physiological effects. As far as is known, humans do not make the exact equivalent of these chemical weapons for themselves. However, some of the components of the immune system, such as interferon and interleukins, could be seen in this light, and there is increasing interest in developing these as medicines.

No one knows how much of the world's biodiversity remains to be discovered by science. Low and high estimates of the total number of species range from four million to 33 million. Of the species that are known to science, only a small fraction has been investigated for medicinal products – just a few hundred out of the 38,000 known plants for instance (even though it is reckoned that half will have some medicinal potential). And researchers tend to look for only one type of drug in a given species – antibiotics from microbes, for instance, or anti-cancer drugs from plants. So even if only one in 10,000 compounds evaluated develops into a drug, the pharmaceutical industry will never exhaust the natural world as a source of new drugs.

But researchers need some guideposts to rummaging in nature's medicine cabinet. Many look to ethnobotany – the study of the folkloric use of plants – for guidance. The opium poppy is probably the best-known example of folk medicine turned to modern use. The plant has been used for at least 5000 years for its powerful analgesic properties. Its two main active components, morphine and codeine, are still important drugs today. And artemesin and its derivative artemether, two new drugs against malaria, come from the sweet wormwood plant which has been used in Chinese medicine for nearly 2000 years.

Another sign that an organism may be worth investigating is toxicity; species that are toxic must, by definition, be making compounds that are biologically active. An obvious example from the plant world is deadly nightshade, from which we get atropine and hyoscine, which are used in eye examination and surgery.

So far, plants and microbes have provided the bulk of medicinal natural products. But there is increasing interest in insects, marine organisms and other groups. There are an estimated 0.5 to 10 million animal species in the oceans, and between one million and 200 million microbes. So far 500 species of marine animal have been shown to have cytotoxic potential – they can kill cancer cells, at least in the test tube. Ecteinascidin-1, a compound from sea-squirts found in Florida, is already being tested in patients with terminal cancer, and there are other potential drugs – from a sponge, a bryozoan, and a sea hare – which have reached a similar stage of development.

Many experts believe that cone snails are the species to go for when it comes to searching out pharmaceutical treasure from the sea. These marine predators have enjoyed extraordinary success throughout 50 million years of evolution, thanks to the venom they manufacture. Venom from an individual species may contain over one hundred different biologically active peptides. These peptides appear to target cell-surface receptors – which, as was explained in Chapter 1, is one of the main modes of drug action – and ion channels. One of these cone venom peptides is already in use, in clinical trials, as an analgesic for intractable pain.

The problem with raiding the natural world for new drugs is whether supplies will be able to meet demand. The discovery of taxol, a new anti-cancer drug which comes from the Pacific yew, was widely used as a strong argument for conserving biodiversity. In fact taxol has created something of an environmental dilemma. It needs an astounding 13,500 kg of Pacific yew bark to yield only one kilogram of taxol. Meeting global demand for taxol could wipe out this endangered species. And taxol has proved to be fiendishly difficult to synthesise in the laboratory.

There are two ways to meet this challenge. At present most taxol is produced by a compromise route; an intermediate compound, baccatin III, is produced from the European yew, which is not on the endangered list. Meanwhile, Japanese biotechnologists have shown that promising amounts of taxol can be obtained using cells from the yew grown in the laboratory (more about cell culture in Chapter 11). Growing cells does not require the destruction of the tree. Further, plant pathologist Gary Strobel of Montana State University has discovered that fungi living on many species of yew also produce taxol. These could also be grown in culture to produce the drug.

Despite these difficulties, the natural world will continue to be a key resource for the pharmaceutical industry. However, the political and economic aspects of 'drug prospecting' are changing, thanks mainly to the UN Convention on Biodiversity. First drafted during the Rio Earth Summit in

1992, the Convention has now been signed by over 160 member states of the United Nations.

Article 15 of the Convention recognises each country's 'sovereign right' over its genetic resources, which includes natural products from which new drugs could be developed. This marks a change from the old understanding that genetic resources were the 'heritage of mankind'. Until recently, casual collection of soil samples or plants by pharmaceutical company employees was the norm when they were on holiday in a foreign country. They would bring them back to the lab to see if they could find any interesting new lead compounds.

If researchers want to go drug prospecting today in the tropical rainforests (or anywhere else for that matter), they have to do it in collaboration with local scientists. Article 19 of the Convention says that the host country has to benefit from such ventures, if they lead to the successful development of a drug or any other product. Pharmaceutical companies rely on natural resources originating in developing countries, and these probably account for a significant proportion of their annual earnings; if the Convention works as it is designed to, the nations who 'own' the resources stand to gain a share of the companies' profits.

It sounds good; but the issue of just compensation is turning out to be a tricky one. Governments 'own' the resources but it is usually indigenous people who have invested the time and effort in them, and have the vital knowledge of ethnobotany which guides Western scientists in their research. In many countries the interests of government and indigenous people diverge; money may be channelled into the wrong hands and unscrupulous politicians could even use Article 19 to deprive people of their land and resources, arguing that these belong to the nation as a whole.

If the Convention is going to work to the benefit of both sides, agreements should perhaps be drawn up on a case-by-case basis. In Costa Rica, for example, the government has licensed its national diversity institute INBio to feed back a proportion of the income it gets from private (and non-exclusive) deals with drug companies for conservation of the country's natural resources. There are similar set-ups in Australia, Nigeria and other central African countries. And an agreement set up between INBio and pharmaceutical giant Merck over development of local botanical sources has been held up to the rest of the industry as a model of how these things should be done.

But such arrangements would not be appropriate in countries with many ethnic groups or with a large indigenous population, according to Maurice Iwu, a Nigerian chemist and expert on development and conservation. In such countries, traditional healers and their communities might need to be central to such agreements – a principle adopted by the US company Shaman Pharmaceuticals.

Some countries have even developed this idea to stop any 'interference' in their resources by foreign countries. In India, a national drug company, the Arya Vaidhya Pharmacy (AVP), is developing the anti-stress drug jeevani from a plant that grows in the Agasthiyar Hills of Kerala State. AVP will give the Kani tribe $25,000 for sharing their traditional knowledge of jeevani, and for cultivating and supplying the plants.

. . . and the other 50 per cent come from the chemical industry

Around the turn of the century, Ehrlich had the idea of exploiting the growing chemical industry for medicines. At the time, the most successful products of the chemical industry (launched in Germany in the 1800s) were dyes, which were used not just on textiles, but as stains in microscopy. Peering down a microscope, Ehrlich saw that the dye Trypan Red was absorbed by trypanosome parasites, which cause a number of diseases including sleeping sickness. Later he developed an arsenic-containing compound called Salvarsan as a reasonably effective drug against syphilis.

During the 20th century the chemical industry has grown enormously – particularly with the switch from coal to petroleum as a feedstock in the 1940s. Petroleum contains thousands of organic compounds. And thousands more have been created from them. Many of these have been elaborated to create useful drugs such as anaesthetics and analgesics. The drug discovery programmes of a drug company leave them with vast libraries of such synthetic compounds, which they can always try out against any new target. Half of the world's top 20 best-selling drugs (Table 1) are completely synthetic.

And old drugs are often the best starting points for new drugs. For instance, the original antihistamines which were used to treat hay fever and other allergies had the problem of causing drowsiness – impairing patients' ability to drive and operate machinery. Chemical modification of the original molecule has led to new antihistamines, such as terfenadine (Triludan), which do not cause sedation. And in a clever variation, the drowsiness side effect of the original drugs has been exploited to make a new type of sleeping pill; diphenhydramine (Nytol) is an antihistamine and the drowsiness it induces is used to overcome insomnia.

However, as any organic chemist will tell you, the problem with making new compounds is that it consumes months, if not years, of precious time. (And while a plant or microbe may contain hundreds of ready-made compounds, extracting and identifying them all is equally time-consuming.)

But over the last few years, a radical new way of synthesising new potential drugs has burst onto the drug discovery scene. Known as combinatorial chemistry, it goes against all the traditions of organic chemistry.

In combinatorial chemistry, thousands – or even millions – of compounds are made in one experiment. Generation of, say, 50,000 new compounds a day is now well within the realms of combinatorial chemistry programmes. Each company (and many small new companies specialising in this new branch of chemistry are now springing up) is developing its own strategy. But three basic combinatorial techniques (Figs 2.2–2.5) can be used to illustrate the principle.

Suppose a compound of potential drug use called AB is made by mixing two components – A and B. Chemical bonds form between A and B, creating the compound AB. For example, you can make aspirin, whose chemical name is acetylsalicylic acid, by mixing acetyl chloride (A) with salicylic acid (B). Then there are a few standard chemical manipulations to carry out – isolating AB from the mixture which contains A and B, purifying it and so on. In traditional chemistry, you might then go on to make a related compound A1B1 by mixing A1 and B1. This would take as long as making AB. In the simplest form of combinatorial chemistry, you would make – say – 25 compounds of the AB type at once by using an array of tiny wells to mix the components in (Fig. 2.2). Each row contains a different type of component A; row one contains A1, row two A2, and so on. And each column contains a different type of B – with B1 in column 1 down to B5 in column 5. Now each well must contain a different pair of A and B components. The top left-hand well contains A1 and B1 because it is in the first row and the first column. The bottom right-hand well contains A5 and B5, as it is in the fifth row and the fifth column. You can see how this technique might lend itself to automatation. A robot arm could add the components to the wells, for example, and carry out routine chemical manipulations to extract and purify the resulting AB type compounds.

This arrangement starts to get rather impractical if you want to make hundreds of compounds at one go. But there is a way of condensing the process by putting a mixture rather than a single compound into each well.

	B1	B2	B3	B4	B5
A1	A1B1	A1B2	A1B3	A1B4	A1B5
A2	A2B1	A2B2	A2B3	A2B4	A2B5
A3	A3B1	A3B2	A3B3	A3B4	A3B5
A4	A4B1	A4B2	A4B3	A4B4	A4B5
A5	A5B1	A5B2	A5B3	A5B4	A5B5

Fig. 2.2. Combinatorial chemistry – simple array. Each of five wells in a row receives a different type of A component, and the wells in the columns receive the corresponding B component. The different A and B components react on mixing to form a set of AB compounds, one per well, from A1B1 to A5B5.

In traditional chemistry, this approach usually ends in tears – the more organic compounds you put together in one vessel, the more likely you are to end up with an intractable black tar. However Glaxo Wellcome, the world's biggest pharmaceutical company, has shown that this approach can work – if the A and B components are carefully chosen, and if there is a systematic way of tracking down what each well contains.

The researchers created a 'library' of 1600 AB type compounds by mixing 40 different A and B components in every possible combination, but in a structured way. First they took an array of 40 wells. Into each one a *single* A component (A1 up to A40) and a mixture of all the B components was dispensed. So each well contained a mixture of 40 different AB compounds. A single well was called a sub-library and it was identifiable by the kind of A component it contained (rather like having a group of books all on the same subject, where the subject is the A component). The mixture of compounds was different in each of the 40 wells. Together, they made up all 1600 possible AB compounds and were called the A series of sub-libraries (Fig. 2.3).

Then a second array of mixtures was created. This time each well contained a single B component and the mixture of all the A components. This second lot of 40 wells was the B series of sub-libraries – and duplicated the total of all 1600 possible AB combinations. So instead of using 1600 single wells, we have reduced the number to only 80 (40 in each series of sub-libraries).

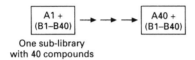

One sub-library
with 40 compounds

'A' series of 40 sub-libraries–containing total of 1600 compounds

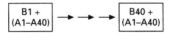

'B' series of 40 sub-libraries–containing total of 1600 compounds

Fig. 2.3. Combinatorial chemistry – using libraries. Each well is a 'sub-library' containing a mixture of 40 different compounds. The A series (top) consists of 40 different sub-libraries, each containing a different A component (A1 to A40) and a mixture of all 40 B components. The B series (bottom) is made in a similar way, with different B components and a mixture of all the A components. Each series contains all 1600 possible combinations of AB compounds (40 wells each with 40 compounds).

The beauty and economy of this system comes out in the screening process. Screening is a quick way of testing potential drug compounds for activity. Suppose we are looking for an enzyme inhibitor. There are chemicals which you can add to the wells, along with the target enzyme, which will give a rapid colour change if the compound binds to the enzyme. Suppose this mixture is added into all 40 wells and gives a 'hit' in the 3rd well of the A series and in the 22nd well of the B series. This shows straight away that the compound A3B22 binds the target and is worthy of further investigation. Hits that have gone into development by this technique include potential anti-psychotic and anti-arthritic drugs.

However, only certain chemical compounds are suitable for synthesis in solution arrays. If you want to build up more complex compounds, using more than one chemical reaction, then the array method becomes rather impractical. The other main type of combinatorial chemistry is known as solid phase synthesis, and comes from an idea developed by Nobel Prize winner Bruce Merrifield as a way of synthesising peptides.

The chemical bond which joins two amino acids together to build up a peptide chain is known as an amide bond. In biological systems, it is made under the influence of enzyme action. In the laboratory, amide bonds can be created between two amino acids, to create a simple peptide. But making peptides of five or more amino acids becomes difficult by the conventional solution chemistry described above. The required peptide is difficult to

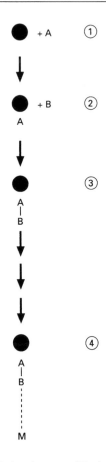

Fig. 2.4. Combinatorial chemistry – solid phase synthesis. (1) A resin bead reacts with amino acid A. (2) After processing, A is linked to the bead, then reacts with B. (3) In a repeat of step 2, a dipeptide AB is now linked to the bead. (4) After 11 more cycles, a string of 13 amino acids, A to M, is now linked to the bead.

separate from a complex mixture of side products (amino acids are chemically quite reactive and will create bonds other than the required amide bond with one another).

Merrifield hit on the idea of linking the first amino acid in the chain to a solid polymer support, which comes in the form of resin beads (Fig. 2.4). This first amino acid, with its bead anchor, could then be linked to the next. Any excess chemicals or impurities could easily be washed off the beads before a third amino acid was added, and so on. In this way Merrifield and

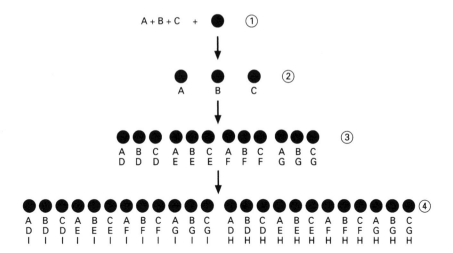

Fig. 2.5. Combinatorial chemistry – 'split and mix' solid phase synthesis. (1) Resin bead reacts with three different amino acids A, B and C. (2) The result is a mixture of beads with either A. B or C attached. (3) The beads are split into four lots and put into four vessels containing amino acids D, E, F and G respectively. The reaction gives four sets of three dipeptides – 12 in all. (4) After mixing the beads are split into two lots, and put into two vessels, one containing amino acid H, one containing amino acid I. Now there are 24 tripeptides – from only three chemical reactions.

other chemists were able to build up peptides of up to 100 amino acids, several of which have been developed as drugs, such as vaccines for malaria and other diseases.

Solid phase synthesis lends itself to automation, and it was not long before peptide synthesisers – arrangements of valves, pumps and tubes which were computer programmable – came on to the market. The technique is also ideal for combinatorial chemistry – making several peptides at once. The method which is currently most used is known as 'split and mix' (Fig. 2.5). In the first stage, you take three pots of beads and anchor amino acids A, B and C respectively to them. Then mix the beads up, split them into four lots and react them with a second amino acid – D, E, F or G. Now you have beads containing every possible combination of A, B, C, D, E, F, and G (12 peptides in all). Mix them again, and react with a third amino acid, H or I, and you will end up with 24 tripeptides in just three chemical steps. The more amino acids are used at each stage, and the more stages are used, the bigger is the mixture of amino acids that is generated. Some companies make literally millions of different peptides in this way. Beads which are found to be active in assays can be identified using microscopic techniques similar to those used in identifying cells. Sometimes chemists make a second compound known as a 'tag' alongside the peptide. The tag is used to identify the peptide of interest after assay, because sometimes the amount of peptide is too small to identify on its own. The tag is a chemical which is easier to identify.

The only drawback with using peptides is that they are not always useful drugs; they are broken down in the gut, and even if given by injection they are sometimes too large to enter the tissues where their target is. But solid phase synthesis, although it originated with peptides, is now being adapted to suit the synthesis of other pharmacologically active compounds.

The first drugs developed through combinatorial chemistry are now well along the road to the marketplace. In 1993, Pfizer identified a lead compound for preventing atherosclerosis, the 'furring up' of arteries that leads to heart disease (of which more in Chapter 5) using conventional chemistry. Then, with combinatorial technology, they created more than a thousand analogues, of which several were up to 100 times more potent than the lead. The intriguing aspect of the project is that they made 900 compounds before these exciting new leads emerged. With conventional chemistry this would have been too time-consuming, and the project would have long since been abandoned. Now the candidate drug is in clinical trials. Another example comes from Eli Lilly, who had a lead compound for migraine which was not going to be specific enough. With combinatorial chemistry, they could rapidly refine the structure of the lead to get a 'cleaner' compound which is also now in human trials.

Computer graphics aid drug discovery

These days chemists can discover new drug leads without needing to step into the laboratory, thanks to a technique called X-ray crystallography and sophisticated computer graphics.

X-ray crystallography was developed in 1912 by father-and-son team William and Lawrence Bragg. It involves firing a beam of X-rays at a crystal of a substance (the Braggs began with simple salts like sodium chloride). The X-rays interact with atoms in the crystal in and get knocked off course, emerging from the crystal in a direction different from the way they entered it. If the crystal is surrounded by X-ray film, the emerging rays create a pattern of spots on it. Mathematical analysis of this pattern allowed the Braggs to build up a picture of the inner arrangement of sodium and chloride ions within the crystal.

In the 1930s, British scientist Dorothy Hodgkin began to apply X-ray crystallography to the analysis of biological molecules to obtain their three-dimensional structures. She cracked the structure of penicillin in 1945 and vitamin B_{12} in 1956, while Max Perutz, working in Cambridge, worked out the first structure of a protein, haemoglobin, around the same time. But undoubtedly the most important structure ever solved by crystallography was that of DNA. Much of the actual crystallography for this breakthrough was carried out by Rosalind Franklin, working at Kings College London with Maurice Wilkins. However, it was Francis Crick and James Watson, based in Cambridge, who put the structure together and published it in 1953.

Today the three-dimensional structures of hundreds of different proteins (and remember, these are the targets of most drugs) are known, along with those of many small organic molecules. If you bring the computer images of a target, such as an enzyme, and a potential drug molecule together on the screen you can see how the two interact – saving weeks, and maybe months, of time ploughing through laboratory screens. Most drug companies now have computer-based libraries of compounds which they can scan against target structures.

So-called computer-aided drug design has played an important role in bringing a new type of AIDS drug, the protease inhibitors, onto the market. Drugs which can hit any part of the life-cycle of the human immunodeficiency virus (HIV) will be potentially effective against AIDS (more on this in Chapter 3). HIV protease is the enzyme the virus uses to process the proteins it needs to infect new cells. If HIV protease is inhibited, the virus particles become non-infective.

The structure of HIV protease was solved in 1989 by three separate teams of crystallographers, two in the US and one at Birkbeck College in London. Its active site is an elongated cavity flanked by two flexible flaps which close around the substrate (HIV protein) when it binds. If the cavity could be blocked by a molecule of the right shape, then the life-cycle of HIV would be interrupted.

In 1990, Rene DesJarlais and her team at the University of California discovered one such molecule in their computer database of molecular images. On screen bromoperidol was a selective inhibitor of HIV protease. Bromoperidol is a relative of haloperidol, a drug used in the treatment of schizophrenia. The search took ten hours; it could have taken months of laboratory time to come up with the same results.

Bromoperidol failed the next stage of development, however. The concentrations needed to have an effect on HIV protease in cell-based tests would have been too toxic for use in humans. But the research sparked off the search for other compounds like bromoperidol, but with more activity at lower concentrations. Recently four HIV protease inhibitors have been licensed for use in people with HIV/AIDS. They reduce viral load in patients and boost the activity of the immune system (and are further discussed in the next chapter).

From test tubes to humans – the story of pre-clinical development

Lead compounds that show genuine promise when they are screened for biological activity will get promoted to the status of candidate drugs. They then enter the next stage – pre-clinical development – and the company will apply for a patent on the compound. Now the clock begins ticking. The company has just 20 years to get the drug onto the market and make enough money to justify the sums invested in its development.

A multidisciplinary team swings into action; their programmes usually overlap to a certain extent, to save time. So the chemists will be scaling up production, while the pharmacologists conduct toxicity tests in animals. But they do not run completely parallel to one another to avoid wasting resources. The company will not want to start making kilogram quantities of a drug that turns out to makes rats' tails drop off (a property which test-tube experiments do not reveal of course). The tasks in front of the team are clear – the company must be able to supply the drug, and has to satisfy the regulatory authorities as to its quality, safety and efficacy.

Making drugs into medicines

The chemists in the team have the job of turning tiny quantities of a drug molecule into millions of pills, patches, or injection-ready ampoules. Before they start thinking big – scaling up from lab to factory scale – they will need to confer with the pharmacologists about the type of molecule they are dealing with. Until now, all that has been important is whether the candidate drug might act against its target. Now questions about its bioavailability need to be addressed to get the formulation and dose right.

The chemists will start making up pills and other formulations in the laboratory. For this the drug will probably be mixed with other materials, known as excipients, which have various functions such as helping form the mixture into pills, or disguising a bitter taste. Look on a packet of painkillers, for example, where excipients such as starch and sorbitol will probably be listed.

Just as important are tests to assess the lifetime of pills and other formulations in the pharmacy or bathroom cabinet. Like foods, medicines have expiry dates, and these are printed on the pack. The chemists also have to consider how well the medicine will perform if it is being shipped to a tropical country.

Meanwhile, other chemists in the team will be starting to look at how to scale up production. As we saw earlier, drugs that come originally from natural products can be manufactured from their original source or they may be synthetic copies. There is a lot to be said for letting nature do the chemistry, where this is practical. But the yield of drugs from plants is variable, harvesting and extraction may be difficult and – as has been discussed – there may be conservation issues at stake.

Biotechnology may play an important role in drug production. The bacteria and fungi which naturally produce antibiotics can be grown in vast numbers in the laboratory, in a process known as fermentation (a term often applied to the production of alcohol from sugar and yeast, but also applicable to many other substances). The conditions under which the fermentation is carried out can often be manipulated so that antibiotic yields are far in excess of those found in nature. And, increasingly, fermentation-type processes involve growing plant cells to obtain their products; the anti-cancer drugs vincristine and vinblastine, from the rosy periwinkle, are made in this way. Then there is genetic engineering, a specialised biotechnology technique in which the products of human genes are manufactured in animal, microbial or plant cells. (This will be discussed more fully in Chapter 11.)

Often, though, the drug will have to be produced on a large scale by synthetic chemistry. Modern drugs may involve up to 15 different synthetic stages. There will usually be several different routes to the drug molecule. The route of choice depends upon factors such as the availability and expense of raw materials, the purity and yield of the final products, and the safety of the process.

Once a method of synthesis and a formulation have been decided on, scale-up studies can start. The company will not start building a factory – or turning an existing factory over to the production of a new drug – just on the basis of being able to make, say, a kilogram of the material. Instead, the chemists will go up in stages – 100 grams to a kilogram, then to 10 kilograms and so on. During all this, they will have specific targets to meet – the toxicologists will want enough to feed to, say, 100 mice over a period of several months, or high quality supplies will be needed for clinical trials. The full scale-up project will probably proceed in parallel with the clinical trials – after all, no one wants to commit themselves to a factory turning out millions of pills if it turns out that the new drugs does not actually work in humans.

Safety matters

Screening tests a potential drug's efficacy. But the very simplicity of the way in which a screen is set up – drug meets target – means that it tells you nothing about any potential harmful effects within a human body. For this, you have to test the drug in animals. Usually two species are used: a small animal such as a rat, hamster or mouse, and a larger one, such as a dog or even a primate (baboon or monkey).

Many different types of toxicology test are demanded by the regulatory authorities before a drug is allowed onto the market. First, and most obvious, are tests of acute toxicity which assess the likelihood of a dose of the drug actually killing you. Small groups of animals are given increasing doses of the drug until either it kills them, or the dose is unrealistically enormous. This establishes the lethal dose. Should this be less than five times the therapeutic dose, the drug will probably be thrown out at this stage (because it would be too dangerous in overdose if it ever got onto the market). But if it looks particularly promising in other ways, the chemists will try to modify it, editing out the molecular feature that may be causing the toxicity. Lethal dose studies form the basis for studies of chronic toxicity. These are especially important for drugs that may be consumed over a period of years, such as contraceptives or a treatment for high blood pressure.

Many drugs also have to be tested to see if they might cause cancer. Here the initial tests do not involve animals, but are done on either bacteria or mammalian cells to see whether they damage their DNA. Substances that do damage DNA are known as mutagens. Many, but not all, of these will be carcinogens. Strongly mutagenic drugs will also be rejected at this stage, although if they are really promising, the chemists may try to modify them.

Since thalidomide, tests have also to be done on pregnant animals to see if potential drugs have effects on reproduction – ranging from impaired fertility to behavioural and other defects in the offspring. And drugs which are destined for use on the skin or eyes will generally be tested for adverse effects in rabbits.

Some people argue that tests in animals cannot tell us about the effects of drugs in humans. There is some truth in this and of course, as we shall see, the drugs are tested in humans before being allowed onto the market. It has also been suggested that animal experiments could be replaced by alternatives – like the Ames test, which evaluates compounds for their mutagenicity in bacteria. No one actually likes doing animal tests and in Britain, at least, they are governed by strict laws.

According to the Animals Act (1986) people doing experiments on animals must be competent, the premises where the experiments are done must be properly staffed and equipped, and the benefits of the research should outweigh the distress involved to the animals. The design of an animal experimentation programme is only approved if it uses the minimum number of animals, and uses alternatives wherever possible.

To be realistic, most of these experiments do involve a degree of suffering, but analgesics and anaesthetics can be used to minimise this. To monitor the Act, Home Office inspectors can – and do – visit pharmaceutical laboratories, sometimes unannounced.

Animal experiments are time-consuming, costly, and turn public opinion against medical research and the pharmaceutical industry. One of the main reasons for the introduction of the Act was to provide a framework for the development of alternatives. These are based on the 'Three Rs' principle introduced by Rex Burch and William Russell in their classic book *The Principles of Humane Experimental Technique* published in 1959.

The Three Rs are reduction, refinement and replacement. Reduction means trying to minimise the numbers of animal experiments by, for example, harmonising regulations so that you do not have to repeat animal experiments for a drug to be approved for use in a new country. Refinement refers to extracting the maximum amount of information from the minimum number of experiments. And there are many possible replacements – from the use of cells, tissues and organ slices to computer models.

Take the notorious Draize test, in which potentially irritating chemicals are dripped into a rabbit's eyes to see whether they attack the cornea. The molecular basis of the irritation is the degradation of a protein molecule found in the eye. The effect can be reproduced in a test tube; a solution of the same protein will turn cloudy when exposed to the irritating chemical. A similar 'alternative' test is the LAL test (lymphocyte amoebocyte lysate) assay. Some compounds produce fever as a side effect (because of trace impurities they contain). The traditional test involves injecting it into an animal to see if it runs a temperature. But blood cells from the horseshoe crab form a clot in a test tube with such fever-inducing drugs. The test does not harm the crab, which can be returned to the sea after giving the blood sample.

Another interesting development is the COMPACT (Computer Optimised Molecular Parametric Analysis of Chemical Toxicity) system, developed by David Lewis and his team at the University of Surrey in the UK. Like computer-aided drug design, discussed earlier, this is based upon the X-ray crystal structure of proteins – this time a group of liver enzymes called cytochrome P_{450}. These are responsible for the metabolic breakdown of drugs; by looking at the structure of a potential drug together with that of P_{450} on the computer screen, you can tell if the enzyme will be able to handle it. COMPACT has already been used to screen many compounds for toxicity and compares favourably – 70 to 80 per cent agreement – with similar tests in animals.

None of these alternative tests is yet allowed as a substitute for animal experiments. That has to wait until regulatory authorities worldwide become convinced that they are as reliable and informative as the corresponding test in an animal. But already the use of alternatives has cut down on the number of animals used to test drugs; they are used as a preliminary 'screen' before moving into animals. Drugs which fail the screen are rejected and never need be tested in animals.

Absorption, metabolism and excretion studies – known collectively as pharmacokinetics – are also done in animals. To find out the journey of the drug molecule from the point of administration – as was described for the aspirin molecule at the start of the last chapter – a radioactively labelled version of the drug is used. This means that one of its atoms is given a radioactive tag. If the distribution of radiation in the animal's body – and its appearance in the urine – is measured over a period of time, then a picture of how the body handles the drug can be built up.

Human testing times – clinical trials

Once sufficient animal testing has been done – and if the results are satisfactory – the candidate drug can be tested in humans. For instance, if the drug has been tested for 15 days in two species, you are allowed to give one to three single doses to humans. To give a longer course of treatment – say up to three months – six months of animal testing is required.

Clinical trials are complex, expensive and time-consuming. Only one in ten candidate drugs entering this stage will emerge as a medicine that can take its place on the pharmacy shelves. It is a time of great excitement – and great risk. The company may enjoy the satisfaction of seeing its investment finally pay off – or it may lose millions of dollars. As trials progress, results are published in medical journals, and may be picked up by the media, giving future consumers of the drug perhaps the first hints of what may soon be on offer for them. Clinical trials, worldwide, are divided into four distinct phases, lasting in total between five and ten years.

Healthy volunteers step forward – phase I clinical trials

However desperate patients might be for a new medicine – a drug against AIDS or a new cancer therapy for example – they usually have to wait until it has been tested in healthy people. These so-called non-patient volunteers often work for the company, but other people such as medical students are often recruited. This recruitment is usually done fairly discreetly – no widespread advertising, or notices in newspapers, for example. On the other hand, a direct approach to a potential volunteer is also frowned on. The aim is to get well-motivated people involved, where financial gain is not the primary aim. The volunteers do get paid for their time and trouble, but the payments are not usually large, and the clinical trials team prefer to have people who are already in employment, to whom the cash will not make much difference.

Up to 100 people take part in a phase I clinical trial. Usually the volunteers are men aged between 18 and 65. Until recently women of child-bearing age were often excluded, because of worries about the impact of an untested drug on any possible foetus. So were the over-65s because, as discussed in Chapter 1, many drugs have greater side effects on older people. Children are never used in phase I clinical trials, and nor are prisoners.

In fact, women and the elderly consume more drugs than men of the age group employed in the phase I trials. In recognition of this mismatch, clinical trials teams now make an effort to recruit women and the over-65s to phase I trials of drugs that are likely to be used most in these patient groups.

There is far more to being in a phase I clinical trial than just taking increasing doses of a new drug. The aim is to see how the human body handles the drug, so volunteers must expect to give many blood and urine samples, and have tests of liver and kidney function. Although the doctors supervising the trials will be on the lookout for toxic effects that have been seen in animals – skin rash, for example – there is always the chance that some unexpected effects will occur when the potential drug is first used in humans. The volunteers' hair could turn green, for example, or there could be psychological effects such as depression or hyperactivity. Really serious side effects are rare, and there are no reports of anyone dying as a result of being in a phase I clinical trial. Even so, only half of all potential drugs make it as far as phase II. By this stage the research team has built up a dossier of data on where the drug goes in the body, its toxicity, how long it stays in the system, and how the body gets rid of it.

Testing medicines on patients – phase II clinical trials

People suffering from the disease the candidate drug is intended for will now be recruited to test it out. Up to 500 patients get involved at this stage – often contacted through specialist clinics in teaching hospitals. Although the team will still be interested in all the factors they investigated in phase I – how the body handles the drug, in short – their main focus of attention is whether the drug can treat disease. The healthy volunteers did not, of course, have the disease, so this is the first opportunity the researchers have to see whether the drug actually works as intended. They will look for the dose required to produce some therapeutic effect, and work out the therapeutic index – the safety margin between the minimum effective dose and the higher dose that starts to produce some adverse effects. If all goes well at this stage, the drug can then be taken to a bigger patient population in phase III clinical trials.

Make or break time – phase III clinical trials

Any potential drug that gets this far is a good candidate for making it onto the market and giving some benefit to patients. But demonstrable benefit in 500 patients does not really justify offering the drug to thousands, or even millions, of people. The trial needs first to be scaled up and this is what happens in phase III, where between one thousand and three thousand patients get involved. As millions of dollars of investment ride on a good outcome to a phase III trial, the way it is designed and carried out is crucial.

A key factor is selection of patients for the trial. Obviously they have to be suffering from the disease the drug is meant to treat, but just how ill should they be? Sometimes a phase III trial is carried out using very sick patients – the rationale being that this is maybe more ethical. In a sense, the terminally ill who have tried everything else have nothing left to lose.

But using very sick patients in a phase III clinical trial has obvious drawbacks. They are – to put it brutally – more likely to die, despite the best efforts to treat them, than less ill patients are. So the success rate of the treatment could be disappointingly low.

The next factor to be considered is what to measure – also known as the clinical end-point. This could be as crude as whether the patient lives or dies. Or it may be a laboratory measurement such as how the number of white blood cells increases over a period of time, or a clinical measurement such as fall in blood pressure. Whatever is chosen it is important that it is a good indicator of the condition which the drug is meant to treat.

The way the trial is carried out is also vitally important. The 'gold standard' in clinical research is the double-blind random crossover trial. The patients are divided into two groups, roughly equal in number and similar in age, sex, severity of illness and other relevant factors. The patients are assigned randomly to their group, by a computer. One group gets the new drug, the other – known as the control group – gets either an existing treatment for the condition, or an inactive treatment known as a placebo. Patients are often given placebo if the condition is not life-threatening. Otherwise it is considered more ethical to offer some treatment, rather than none at all.

The drug company has to design placebo pills or injections that look the same, and are delivered in the same way, as the candidate drug. The same goes for any existing treatment that is being used in the control group.

Neither the doctor or nurse administering the treatment should know whether their patients are in the treatment group or the control group. Nor do the patients know which group they are in. This is to prevent any bias. For instance, if the doctor knew who was in the treatment group, he or she might – maybe unconsciously – give those patients more attention, and this could affect the outcome of the trial. Similarly, if patients knew they were on the drug, they might say – or even convince themselves – that they felt better, to please the doctors (and this would have to be recorded as part of the data, even though it probably would not be the clinical end-point).

Being in a phase III clinical trial tends to benefit most of the patients enrolled in it – even those in the control group. It is up to the clinical trial team to work out how much of this benefit is actually due to the candidate drug. All the patients in the trial may well benefit from the extra medical attention they are getting, which of course has to be the same for each group. Then there will be improvements in the control group – either from being given an existing treatment, which presumably is known to have at least some benefit, or from the placebo. That patients often get better when given 'sugar pills' (placebos) is well known in medicine, although how the placebo response happens is not at all well understood. In the trial any improvement the treatment group shows over and above that shown by the control group is assumed to be due to the candidate drug.

In a crossover trial the patients switch groups halfway through the trial. Both groups should show a similar pattern of response to the candidate drug, which is in effect being tested on the whole group – giving twice as much data as if there were no crossover. It is also more ethical – all the patients have had a chance to receive the new drug. Occasionally, a candidate drug gives such good results that it would be unethical not to offer it to all the patients. This happened recently in the trial of a new drug called ReoPro, which decreases the 'stickiness' of the blood. It was given to patients with angina before they underwent surgery to unblock their coronary arteries – a procedure which carries a risk of blood clot formation. ReoPro gave such good results that the trial was stopped early, so all the patients could have a chance to take it.

Sometimes a trial may also be stopped prematurely if it becomes obvious that the candidate drug is actually harming the patients on it. For instance, in 1993 Centocor, a US biotechnology company, had to halt trials on a drug meant to treat septic shock, a life-threatening condition triggered by overwhelming infection for which there is no effective treatment. Patients in the treatment group showed a higher mortality rate (41 per cent) than those in the placebo group (37 per cent).

Once the trial is over, the results are analysed by medical statisticians to see how good the new drug really is. Sometimes the patients on the treatment may appear to have done better than the controls, but the results are not statistically significant – in other words, they could have arisen by chance. Another drug which was meant to target septic shock, Antril, developed by biotechnology company Synergen, fell at this last hurdle – wiping millions of dollars off the company's shares and sending shock waves through other companies which had invested in this difficult therapeutic area. Antril is a receptor antagonist for interleukin-I (IL-1), one of the key chemicals involved in the body's inflammatory response to infection. In septic shock, inflammation goes into overdrive and causes great damage to the body. Synergen hoped their candidate drug would get inflammation under control by neutralising IL-1. When the results of the phase III clinical trials of Antril were analysed however, they showed that 29 per cent of patients receiving Antril died, compared with 34 per cent on placebo. At least the change was in the right direction, but given the numbers of patients involved, the statisticians declared that the results were not significant enough and the drug was not given the much-desired licence. Needless to say Synergen lost millions, and had to go back and design another clinical trial.

Another option in cases like this, where benefits of a new treatment seem to be small, is to carry out a statistical procedure known as a meta-analysis. This involves researchers combing through the medical literature for examples of clinical trials on a particular drug. These data can be combined and analysed to simulate the results of a much bigger study.

Meta-analysis played a big part in gaining acceptance for thrombolytic drugs – sometimes known as 'clot busters' – within the medical profession. These are meant to increase the chances of survival after heart attack by dissolving the clot which cuts off the blood supply to the heart muscle (this will be discussed further in Chapter 5). Smaller trials had suggested there were benefits, but these were not statistically significant and emergency care doctors did not include thrombolytic therapy as part of the treatment for their heart attack patients. But when a number of these small trials were combined in a meta-analysis, the results did reach statistical significance. As a result, thrombolytic therapy, though expensive, is now given after heart attack and, increasingly, after a stroke – with the saving of many lives.

Although being in a clinical trial can greatly benefit patients, and trials are essential if new drugs are to get onto the market to help the wider patient population, it can be hard to recruit people to them at this stage. Many trials do not even get off the ground for this reason. In the UK at present, there are 500 clinical trials going on of new cancer treatments. But fewer than five per cent of all cancer patients are involved.

When patients go to a specialist with a potentially life-threatening disease like cancer they expect to be offered the best treatment available at the time. The prospect of joining a clinical trial in which they may be offered no treatment at all, if they end up in the control group, is unacceptable to many – as is the thought that their consultant will not even know what treatment the patient is receiving. At the same time, they know that without their participation the best treatment available – which is what they want to be offered – can never be improved upon.

Patients today are far better informed than they used to be, thanks mainly to the setting up of self-help groups, and better education. Some refuse to enter clinical trials at all; others enter and manipulate the programme to their own ends. For example, groups of AIDS patients in the US formed the pressure group ACT UP to campaign against the use of placebos. Some of those in trials of the drug AZT got together and shared out their drugs so that they would all at least get some AZT, albeit a lower dose than the treatment group would have got. If this happens in a clinical trial, the results are obviously going to be meaningless. If patient participation – or non-participation – problems like this persist, it might be necessary to find alternatives to the classical double-blind trial which are acceptable to the regulatory authorities.

Once all the clinical trials have been completed a massive dossier of data – running to say 40,000 pages – is submitted to the authorities. In the UK this is either the Medicines Control Agency (MCA) or the European Agency for the Evaluation of Medicinal Products (EMEA), and in the US the Food and Drugs Administration (FDA). These authorities scrutinise it and decide whether to give the drug its much-coveted licence.

Life after licensing – phase IV trials and yellow cards

Once a new drug has been licensed, the company does not just abandon it and get on with making the next drug. The medicine is now being field tested in hundreds of thousands of patients and undoubtedly some unexpected side effects which did not show up in the specially selected phase III patients, will occur. There may also be new indications for its use – so the company can get extra mileage from its investment. For instance, once it was discovered that the bacterium *Helicobacter pylori* plays an important role in the development of stomach ulcers, Glaxo was able to develop a new formulation of Zantac which contains an antibiotic.

In phase IV trials, the company recruits a number of doctors and asks them to report back on the experiences of the first 100 or so people to whom they prescribe the new drug. After this, long-term surveillance is carried out via the 'yellow-card' system. If patients experience side effects, then doctors write them up on a yellow card which is forwarded (in the UK) to the Department of Health.

If things go badly wrong, patients may sue the company – and if the case is proven the drug may even be withdrawn from the market. To date around 100 drugs – out of around 6000 currently available – have been banned, including the anti-arthritis drug Opren and the sleeping pill Halcion.

Halcion is triazolam, a short-acting benzodiazepine (a class of tranquilliser). Its use was suspended in the UK in 1991 and a permanent ban imposed in 1993. The reason was that triazolam may cause rebound insomnia – once you stop taking it the sleeplessness returns, and is possibly worse than before – as well as anxiety, depression and other psychiatric symptoms. Currently hundreds of former users are suing manufacturer Upjohn for the damage they allege Halcion has done to their mental health. Upjohn strongly resisted the move to ban Halcion and has taken every possible route of appeal to get the drug reinstated (the drug is still in use in several other countries, however).

The long route from the laboratory bench to the pharmacy shelf is strewn with potential disappointment and failure. But the industry has produced enough winners to make the game worth playing. In particular, it has been responsible for perhaps the biggest medical advance of the 20th century – antibiotics, which are the subject of the next chapter.

3

Fighting infection

We begin our survey of pharmaceutical drugs with medicines that treat infectious disease – from sore throats and flu to TB and AIDS. Anti-infective drugs have been the trail-blazer for the pharmaceutical industry. Penicillin, for example, has probably been the most significant medical discovery of the 20th century. But, as we shall see, the fight against infection is far from over and we still desperately need drugs and vaccines to cope with major killers such as TB, malaria and AIDS.

The continuing world war

The course of human history has been shaped as much by microbes as by politicians, soldiers, and great thinkers such as Aristotle and Darwin. Smallpox alone has probably claimed more lives than any other disease in human history. Typhus among the troops was a deciding factor in Napoleon's retreat from Moscow in 1812, the English Civil War, and many important battles in Europe (World War II was the first major conflict in which more soldiers died in battle than from infectious disease). John Keats, George Orwell, and Vivien Leigh are only a few of the famous figures who have died prematurely of TB. And today the big killers such as AIDS and malaria are devastating the economies of developing countries – with knock-on effects for the rest of the world.

The war against infection will never be over. The latest figures issued by the World Health Organization (WHO) show that in 1995 17 million people – most of them children – died of infectious diseases. Pneumonia topped with list with four million deaths, followed by TB and malaria with 3.1 million deaths each. Cholera, typhoid, and dysentry between them claimed another three million lives, while hepatitis B, HIV/AIDS and measles were each responsible for a further million deaths. Finally a million deaths were from tetanus, whooping cough or intestinal worms.

The pattern of infectious disease throughout the world changes constantly – not least because new diseases emerge from time to time, and old ones come back. The WHO estimates that there have been at least 30 new diseases over the last 20 years. Some of the more important are Ebola fever which appeared in 1976, AIDS which was first reported in the early 80s, hepatitis C in 1989 and Legionnaire's disease in 1977. Meanwhile a new strain of Creutzfeldt-Jakob disease (CJD), apparently transmitted from cattle to humans, has emerged in the UK. TB and malaria – two 'old' diseases which were thought to be under control – are on the increase again, and there has been a re-emergence of diphtheria in Eastern Europe.

However, some infectious diseases are on their way out. In 1967 the WHO committed itself to ridding the world of smallpox with a mass immunisation campaign. The last case of smallpox occurred in 1978 – oddly enough in Britain, when medical photographer Janet Parker died after contracting the disease from a laboratory sample. The year before an Ethiopian cook, Ali Mao Moallin, became the last person to catch smallpox in the normal way. In theory, however, smallpox could stage a comeback because stocks of the smallpox virus still exist in research laboratories in the United States and in Russia. In recent years, the WHO Assembly has been discussing whether or not to destroy these stocks, to ensure that the world's population really is safe from its re-emergence. This would be the first deliberate extinction of a natural organism. So far, the virus has had several stays of execution and the current plan is to destroy it on 30 June 1999. The virus 'lives on' in the sense that its genome – the sum of its genetic material – has been sequenced and cloned (for more about genetics and infection, see Chapter 11). So we probably have sufficient knowledge of the virus without having to study it any further.

Guinea worm, a parasitic disease of the tropics, is set to follow smallpox into extinction. Other infectious diseases on the WHO hit-list for eradication are polio, measles, leprosy, whooping cough, and river blindness, a tropical disease caused by a parasitic worm. According to the latest data, the world should be rid of polio by the year 2005. Then, as with smallpox, the WHO will destroy the polio virus itself. Next to go should be measles, by the year 2010.

There are four main factors which determine the current global pattern of infectious disease. Rapid population growth has gone hand in hand with urbanisation; it is estimated that by the year 2000 well over half of the world's population will live in towns and cities, compared to around 40 per cent in 1996. You might think living in a city would mean access to better healthcare, and a higher standard of living. This is not so for most of today's new urban dwellers, most of whom are in developing countries. For them city living means overcrowding, poor hygiene, and poor living conditions, which spell out ideal conditions for the spread of disease. No wonder then, that after many years of decline, tuberculosis is on the increase again in some of the world's capitals such as New York City, London, Paris and Amsterdam. Yes, these are in the developed world – but in the poorer areas of say, New York City, conditions are actually worse than in many a developing country.

Urbanisation also leads to new habitats for microbes. Rubbish dumps for example allow mosquitoes to breed in the small pools of water that collect in discarded aluminium cans, bottle tops, and rubber tyres. Such a scenario probably led to the re-emergence of dengue fever in the mid 1950s. Dengue fever is caused by an arbovirus, which is carried by the mosquito *Aedes aegypti*. It is now classified as one of the world's most dangerous tropical diseases by the WHO, for there is no vaccine and no cure and the number of countries affected has risen from nine to more than 40 since 1970. New Delhi, for instance, has just suffered its worst epidemic of the disease since the 1960s, with 7000 people affected and over 270 dead at the last count.

Changing patterns of land use have brought many microbes into contact with humans for the first time. For example, in the 19th century land clearance for agriculture in parts of Europe and America was followed by reforestation. This type of land turned out to be an ideal habitat for deer. Later, people began to build in these areas, and they became popular spots for a day out in the country. Man and microbe were now on a collision course; deer harbour ticks, which in turn carry the bacterium *Borrelia burgdorferi*. Should the ticks bite a human, they may infect him with this bug, which can cause Lyme disease (named after Old Lyme in Connecticut where the disease was first reported in 1975). Lyme disease is characterised by weakness, headache and joint pain. It can be difficult to diagnose, but the longer it remains untreated the harder it is to cure.

War and political change often lead to breakdown in crucial public health programmes. For many years immunisation programmes have kept the killer disease diphtheria under control around the world. Now, as previously mentioned, it is emerging in the former Soviet Union as an indirect result of the profound changes that have taken place there over the past decade. The epidemic broke out in 1990 and peaked in 1995 when more than 1500 people died. Neighbouring countries did not escape; Finland had reported no cases of diphtheria for 30 years, but had four in 1994, while two

Americans caught it on a visit to the former Soviet Union. Now, thanks to the concerted efforts of aid organisations who organised mass vaccination, the epidemic appears to be in retreat and there has been no further spread to other parts of Europe. But war has hindered the drive to eradicate polio, which was originally set for the year 2000. The aim is to vaccinate every child in the world; this is often not possible in areas of strife. The last case of polio in the Americas was a Peruvian boy who missed out on vaccination when his local clinic was destroyed by guerillas. But sometimes it has been possible to organise temporary ceasefires for polio vaccination; there were such truces between the Tamil Tigers and the Sri Lankan army in 1995 and 1996, and similar 'days of tranquillity' in the Sudan and El Salvador. These 'glimpses of peace', when both sides share a common goal, may do more than help defeat disease, says Harry Hull of the WHO's Global Programme for Vaccines and Immunization. Writing in the journal *Science* Hull comments that the vaccination days may also serve as a valuable tool in the resolution of conflict.

Microbes are no respecters of international boundaries and frontiers and take advantage of increased business and leisure travel, and the growth of world trade, to hitch a lift to new habitats. In 1993 another new disease, Hantavirus pulmonary syndrome, killed 32 people in the United States. Hantavirus, however, is common in the Far East – and had almost certainly been carried to the US by a mouse or rat hiding out in a commercial cargo.

Changing patterns of human health also invite new types of infectious disease. People are living longer all over the world, but the immune system weakens with age making infection more likely. People with AIDS and cancer also have severely compromised immunity. Ironically, some of the most advanced treatments leave the body open to infection. Organ transplant surgery and cancer chemotherapy and radiotherapy all undermine the immune system, while placing lines, catheters and other devices in the body also makes it vulnerable to infection. These factors mean that being admitted to hospital could actually make you ill. The numbers affected by nosocomial infections – the clinical term for an infection acquired in the hospital environment – are rising year on year. Currently septic shock, a potentially fatal condition resulting from overwhelming infection, is the commonest cause of death in the intensive care unit. Not only is this a tragedy for family and friends, it is also a waste of high-tech treatment.

Most worrying of all is the fact that our main weapons against infection, antibiotic drugs, seem to be losing their power, as microbes increasingly develop the ability to resist them. The problem of antibiotic resistance will be discussed more fully in the next section.

How microbes make you ill

Microbes are organisms which are too small to be visible to the naked eye. There are four main categories – viruses, bacteria, fungi and protozoa. (Prions, which are thought to cause diseases such as CJD and kuru in humans, and BSE in cattle, defy categorisation – the best way to describe them is as infectious proteins which, unlike other infective organisms, do not appear to contain either DNA or RNA.)

The majority of the microbes who share our world are harmless – indeed, some are positively beneficial to us. There are microbes in the air, the soil, the food and water we consume and on our bodies. In fact there are as many bacteria on the skin of the human body as there are people on the planet. Microbes are also found in the stomach, nose, mouth and – most of all – in the colon, which is home to over 300 species (a gram of faeces typically contains a thousand billion microbes, most of which are bacteria).

When two organisms, in this case humans and various species of microbes, live in close association, the relationship is known as symbiosis. At best, both parties benefit – a state known as mutualism. For example when staphylococci which live on human skin produce acid secretions, these repel potentially harmful bacteria. In return, the staphylococci benefit from feeding off dead skin cells. It is only when the relationship shifts out of balance, into a state known as parasitism, that we may be harmed by a microbe; such harmful microbes are known as pathogens. When the parasite is growing and actively multiplying the human host is said to be infected – although infection does not necessarily lead to disease.

What makes an innocent microbe into a pathogen? Some microbes such as *Vibrio cholerae*, the bacterium which causes cholera, are born pathogens because they have inherent ability to harm the body – a property known as virulence. Others are like the ordinarily mild-mannered man who becomes an aggressive beast behind the wheel of his car; they turn pathogenic only under certain circumstances. For instance, in AIDS, many normally innocent bacteria and fungi can give rise to lethal infections merely because the body's defences against them have broken down. In some cases sheer numbers make innocent microbes into killers. If the microbial load of a particular species in the body suddenly increases then the infection may take hold. For example, the common yeast *Candida albicans* often overgrows and produces vaginal infections after a woman has taken anti-bacterial drugs. Not only does the drug kill pathogens, it may also wipe out innocent bacteria which would normally keep *Candida* in check.

Once infection is present, it can damage the body in two main ways. First, it may produce a toxin. Many of the microbes which produce diarrhoeal diseases – from cholera to holiday tummy – produce poisons which act on the bowel. The toxin produced by *Corynebacterium diphtheriae* is highly potent. It inhibits protein synthesis – without which the cell cannot function – and one molecule of the toxin is enough to kill a single cell. Diphtheria is often fatal, because the toxin travels around the body, causing damage to tissue in the brain, heart and kidney.

Even without toxins, microbes cause damage when they invade and multiply in the cells and tissues of the body. The infected cells send out chemical signals to the immune system which produces an inflammatory response (the other components of the immune system will be discussed later in this chapter). Cells of the immune system release chemicals such as histamine which have a wide range of physiological effects including redness, pain, swelling, and heat. The mere presence of a microbe in the body may produce fever directly. This may be uncomfortable for the victim, but can ultimately be beneficial as the raised temperature slows down the rate of multiplication of the pathogen.

The body has a number of other defences against pathogens. The skin itself forms a barrier, while tears contain an antimicrobial enzyme called lysosyme. The secretions of the vagina are acidic, creating an unwelcome environment for most microbes, and the gastric juices in the stomach are extremely acidic. Recent research has shown that the skin and the tongue actually contain antibiotic substances which repel infection.

The very young are susceptible to infection because their immune systems are not properly developed, while the old are vulnerable because their bodily defences are in decline. Even your genes can, it seems, determine how likely it is that you will succumb to infection. Scientists working in the Gambia found that people who seemed resistant to malaria had a high level of tumour necrosis factor (TNF), a natural substance produced by the body as part of its armoury against infection. It turned out these people had a different variant of the TNF gene, which allowed them to produce more TNF than the rest of the population.

Once infection does break out, its impact depends upon the setting. A disease may be endemic – present at a steady low level – in a given country, like the common cold in the UK. An epidemic is a sudden increase in a disease over the expected level, such as AIDS and now, many experts agree, TB. A pandemic is an epidemic which affects a large area – either the world itself, or a whole continent. Outbreaks are sudden, unexpected local occurrences of infectious disease, such as the clusters of meningitis or food poisoning that have occurred in the UK over the years.

Successful treatment of infection relies on identifying the microbe responsible. To do this doctors still rely quite heavily on Koch's postulates. Robert Koch (1843–1910) was a German physician who was the first to show that microbes could cause disease. However, the ground was prepared by Joseph Lister, Louis Pasteur and others who showed that getting rid of microbes could lower the incidence of disease.

Koch, who won a Nobel Prize for his work in 1905 and isolated the microbe that causes TB, said that the microbe responsible must be isolated from every case of the disease. Then it should be injected into laboratory animals, which should then show signs of the disease. And finally, the same microbe should be isolated again from the ailing animals. Koch's postulates are not universally applicable however. They do not appear to apply to AIDS, for example, which has led a few scientists to question whether the human immunodeficiency virus (HIV) really causes AIDS. The real reason, however, may have more to do with the difficulty of finding animal models of AIDS, and of other diseases that do not fit Koch's theory.

Bacterial diseases

Only a few of the thousands of bacteria that share our planet cause disease. Quite often bacteria cause diseases that resemble viral diseases: meningitis and pneumonia are two examples. The commonest bacterial infections include sexually transmitted diseases and urinary, throat and chest infections. Bacteria also cause most boils and abscesses.

TB: a global emergency One hundred years ago TB was as much feared as cancer is today – and with good reason, for it was responsible for perhaps one in seven of all deaths in Europe (a figure which is not dissimilar to the current rate of mortality from cancer). Until the 1980s TB was in decline all over the world. Now that encouraging picture has changed and TB is on the march again. In many countries rates of decline have either slowed, or flipped into an actual increase. The trend was first noted in the United States where a study of exposure to TB infection in Navy recruits showed a fall from 6.6 per cent to 3.2 per cent between 1950 and 1964. In 1986, the figure was at an all time low at 1.2 per cent. But in 1990 it had risen to 2.5 per cent – a significant and worrying trend. Now the World Health Organization, which declared TB a 'global emergency' in 1993, predicts a 36 per cent increase in the annual number of new cases worldwide, from 7.5 million in 1990 to 10.2 million in 2000. The reasons for the increase in TB include HIV infection – which predisposes towards TB – migration, poverty and malnutrition, and a decrease in control of the disease.

Around 20 per cent of the world's population is probably infected with the TB organism, *Mycobacterium tuberculosis*. Of these, around 20 million people are estimated to have the disease, and around three million die of it every year. Perhaps one in ten of these will be HIV positive. Rates of TB are around ten times greater in Africa than they are in the US and Western Europe. And there is roughly twice as much TB in Eastern European countries as there is in Western Europe. The worst affected country is India, which has 26 per cent of the world's cases of TB.

M. tuberculosis is an airborne infection. The microbe's remarkable success as a killer can be attributed to the waxy covering around it which makes it hard to kill by disinfectants, as well as giving it the ability to evade the immune system. When it gets into the lungs, it attracts white cells and nodules known as tubercles are formed. Over time – if the immune system does not conquer the infection – these become 'cheesy' and harden. These lesions may show up on a chest X-ray. The infection may then spread around the body. Symptoms include fever, fatigue, weight loss and spitting blood. Treatment is by antibiotics such as isoniazid and rifampicin – usually as a 'cocktail' of two or more drugs which must be taken over a period of some months. The fatality rate is about 15 per cent, if treatment is given. Without treatment, one in two will die.

Surprising new roles for bacteria Bacterial infection can set the scene for the emergence of chronic diseases. In 1982 J. Robin Warren and Barry Marshall of the Royal Perth Hospital found that nearly all their patients with gastritis – a stomach infection that predisposes to the development of ulcers – were infected with the bacterium *Helicobacter pylori*. Furthermore, the infection is found in the majority of people with ulcers. In 1991, Martin Glaser of Vanderbilt University, and other researchers, showed that there is also a link between *H. pylori* and stomach cancer (it was already known that having an ulcer is a risk factor for stomach cancer). Glaser had been studying the health of nearly 6000 Japanese-Americans from the 1960s, taking and freezing blood samples at the start of the project for later analysis. Two per cent of them eventually developed stomach cancer. When their blood was compared with that of men who did not have stomach cancer, Glaser found that men who had been infected with *H. pylori* at the start of the study were six times more likely to have stomach cancer. In 1994, the World Health Organization declared *H. pylori* a Class I carcinogen – the most dangerous rank given to cancer-causing agents. To date, no other bacterium has been awarded this dubious honour.

H. pylori is one of the world's most common infections. Three-quarters of the world's population are infected with it. But only ten per cent of people with the infection go on to develop any disease. The infection is commoner in developing countries; in the UK probably around half of all middle-aged people have *H. pylori*. The infection develops in childhood, and its incidence has been decreasing over the years in industrialised nations – perhaps because of improved standards of hygiene. Gastric cancer, too, appears to be in decline – an observation which firms up the link with *H. pylori*.

It may seem strange that any organism can live in the strong acid conditions of the stomach. But *H. pylori* produces an enzyme called urease, which can neutralise stomach acidity in the niches that it chooses to colonise. It is only found in the gastric epithelium, which lies underneath the layer of mucus that coats the stomach. Once there, it produces a toxin which damages cells.

Drugs such as Zantac have practically abolished major surgery for ulcers; now, in light of knowledge about the role of *H. pylori*, antibiotics such as clarithromycin in conjunction with conventional anti-ulcer medication are regarded as being more effective, at least in the United States. Without antibiotics, ulcers often recur, condemning the patient to a lifetime of medication. With antibiotics, the ulcer disappears within weeks and does not return.

Scientists at University College London have even given antibiotics to a small group of patients with gastric lymphoma, a rare stomach cancer, and found that the tumours shrank in response to treatment. Now some experts would like to eradicate *H. pylori* from the population – in much the same way as smallpox has been wiped out. Vaccines are already being tested with this goal in mind.

Eradication of *H. pylori* could lead to enormous public health benefits, for the bacterium is also implicated in childhood diarrhoeal disease which kills 1.5 million under-fives in Africa each year. It is probably also the cause of indigestion and other chronic digestive complaints which account for ten per cent of GP consultations in the UK.

What is perhaps even more surprising is a potential link between *H. pylori* and cot death, uncovered by Barry Marshall (mentioned above). He noted an unexpectedly high rate of infection in cot death babies. This could explain why parents who lose one child to cot death run a higher risk of losing a second. Eradicating the infection from the whole family could be crucial to solving the problem.

And *H. pylori* also appears to be a factor in the development of heart disease. In a study of nearly 300 patients at two hospitals in Yorkshire reported in 1996, those with diseased coronary arteries were more likely to have *H. pylori* infection than those patients with normal arteries. There is also mounting evidence that another common bacterium, *Chlamydia pneumoniae*, may be implicated in the development of heart disease. (Another *Chlamydia* species, *C. trachomatis*, is the cause of one of the commonest sexually transmitted diseases – an inflammation of the urethra which often leads to female infertility by scarring the Fallopian tubes.) *Chlamydia pneumoniae* is usually responsible for throat and chest infections and nearly everyone gets infected with it at some time.

People with heart disease often have high levels of antibodies to *C. pneumoniae*, suggesting repeated exposure to the organism; moreover diseased arteries show tell-tale signs of the presence of the bacterium in the form of its DNA and proteins. And finally, *C. pnemoniae* itself has been found in tissue grown from diseased arteries by James Summersgill and his team at the University of Louisville, Kentucky. The theory is that atheroma – the fatty deposits that build up in and block the coronary arteries – might be due, in part, to an inflammatory response to infection by *C. pneumoniae*, which may be carried from the alveoli of the lungs in macrophages (white cells that help fight infection) towards sites of irritation in the arteries caused by, say, cigarette smoking.

Experiments in mice show that those infected with *C. pneumoniae* tend to develop atherosclerosis more readily than uninfected animals. The evidence that *C. pneumoniae* is more than an 'innocent bystander' in the chronic inflammatory process that leads to heart disease is mounting. In a small study of heart attack victims, Sandeep Gupta of St George's Hospital, London, gave half a single dose of antibiotics and the other half a placebo. The antibiotic group had two-thirds fewer hospital admissions for angina and other heart problems over the following 18 months, compared with the placebo group.

Fungal diseases

Only 50 out of thousands of fungi produce disease in man. One of these, *Candida albicans*, is a normal inhabitant of the human gut. If this delicate balance is upset – by the use of drugs such as oral contraceptives or antibiotics, say, or if the immune system is depleted as in AIDS, then *C. albicans* may overgrow, giving rise to a condition called candidiasis. This is associated with a wide range of symptoms such as lethargy, food intolerance, headaches, irritable bowel syndrome, vague aches and pains, and abdominal pain. *C. albicans* is also the cause of oral and vaginal thrush, and may produce fatal infection in AIDS patients.

Protozoan diseases

Malaria is the biggest parasitic disease affecting humans. Around half the world's population is at risk of malaria, which infects around 267 million people in 103 different countries. There are 150 million cases of malaria each year and it kills up to two million people, including one million children in Africa alone. Some parts of the world are seeing a resurgence of malaria in recent years. There have been four major epidemics of the disease in India since 1994, and it has returned to Turkey, Azerbaijan and Brazil. Climate change may spread malaria further north than ever before in years to come.

The name malaria means 'bad air' because at one time it was thought that it was caused by air rising from foul marshes. But 100 years ago British physician Ronald Ross, working in Hyderabad, showed that malaria was an infectious disease caused by the protozoan parasite *Plasmodium* which is carried by the *Anopheles* mosquito. When the female mosquito bites a human to take a meal of blood, she transmits the parasite, which first makes its way to the liver. Here it multiplies, and after a variable incubation period passes into the bloodstream, where it invades red blood cells. Rapid multiplication of the parasite destroys the red blood cell; it bursts open and releases the parasites – an event which triggers the familiar symptoms of chills and fever.

Malaria is not the only important tropical disease caused by parasites. Each year there are eight million cases of trypanosomiasis, 12 million of leishmaniasis and 500 million of amoebic dysentery. These may affect mainly people in developing countries, but with the expansion of global travel, more and more people in the West are contracting them from travel abroad; for instance, 2000 people in the UK have contracted malaria each year recently.

Viral diseases

A virus consists of a strand of genetic material – either DNA or RNA – inside a protein coat known as a capsid, which has a helical or icosahedral shape. In addition to this, some viruses are surrounded by an 'envelope' of protein. Viruses lie on the borderline between living and non-living entities. They can only reproduce inside a living cell, by hijacking some of its bio-chemical machinery, but they have their own genes which code for viral proteins. Viruses are always parasitic, and there are around 400 which cause a range of diseases in humans from the common cold, flu and mumps to AIDS, polio and cancer.

Influenza The influenza – or flu – virus is spread through the air on the tiny droplets that are created when people cough or sneeze. There are three strains of flu virus, called A, B, and C and these are classified according to the protein molecules known as antigens which they display on their surfaces. However, the antigens of the A and B strains are capable of such extensive mutation that they are difficult for the immune system to keep up with; this process of rapid change of the virus is known as antigenic shift and it is a major headache for scientists trying to develop vaccines for viral diseases. Antigenic shift occurs almost yearly with strain A of the flu virus. So even though an attack of flu will confer immunity on the host for a while, if a mutated strain comes along the body will not have any natural immunity to it and will succumb again. This is why flu continues to create epidemics and even pandemics on a regular basis. The symptoms of flu – sore throat, fever, aches and pains – come from the death of infected cells in the respiratory system. Flu alone is rarely fatal, but it may set the stage for more serious bacterial infections such as pneumonia which can kill susceptible people such as the elderly and those with weak hearts. The flu pandemic of 1918–1919 killed 20 million people – twice as many as perished in battle during World War One.

Viral haemorrhagic fevers The viral haemorrhagic fevers are among the most frightening diseases known. They are characterised by massive internal bleeding, circulatory shock, and a high fatality rate. There are no vaccines and no cures. The viruses responsible live in animals and are transmitted by insects to humans. In the late 1960s, there was an outbreak of viral haemorrhagic fever in the town of Marburg in Germany among scientists who contracted the virus from cells of Ugandan monkeys they were working with.

Another outbreak – of Ebola fever in Zaire and Sudan in 1975 – infected over a thousand people, killing about half of them, including many of the Belgian nurses and doctors working in hospitals in the affected areas. Viral haemorrhagic fevers are particularly worrying because they tend to erupt unexpectedly whenever humans move into new areas, or when living conditions deteriorate and the viruses jump to new animal reservoirs. No one knows where and when another Ebola might emerge, and if it could be contained. It is entirely possible that tourists could bring it back to Europe or North America given the increase in the numbers opting for adventure holidays and exotic travel.

AIDS The origin of the human immunodeficiency virus (HIV) is unknown. However, many researchers think it may have arisen in Africa in the 1950s when the original virus jumped species, from monkey to human.

HIV undermines the immune system, leading to AIDS (Acquired Immune Deficiency Syndrome) which makes the body vulnerable to a range of infections and other diseases that are characteristic of the condition. One of these is a rare cancer, Kaposi's sarcoma, which arises from blood vessels in the skin, and appears as huge purple nodules. It was reports of Kaposi's sarcoma in homosexual men in the early 1980s that alerted the medical community to the fact that something unusual was going on. Today over 21 million people worldwide are infected with HIV, making it the greatest pandemic of the second half of the 20th century. More than 90 per cent of AIDS cases are in developing countries.

HIV is transmitted during exposure of the victim's bloodstream to infected body fluids (such as blood and semen) via sexual intercourse, blood transfusion, needlestick injury, or from mother to foetus. Understanding how HIV infection occurs and how it progresses to AIDS has been one of the most taxing research challenges of the century. The immune system, which is HIV's target, consists of a complex network of white blood cells and chemical messengers. When challenged it mounts a sophisticated response, which is still incompletely understood. Many major breakthroughs in the science of immunology were still to be made when AIDS was first identified in 1981. AIDS research has consumed billions of dollars and dominated the careers of thousands of talented scientists. But it is only now that the research is translating into proven clinical benefit – thanks to new insights into the nature of the virus, and how it interacts with its human host.

HIV is a retrovirus: its genetic material is RNA rather than DNA. It infects a range of white blood cells, the most important of which appears to be the CD4 or T helper cells. These are so-called because they bear molecules of a protein called CD4 on their surface. Put simply, CD4 cells trigger antibody production as part of the immune response to infection. Antibodies are protein molecules which 'lock on' to 'foreign' molecules on invading microbes and so on and help destroy them.

The envelope of HIV is studded with molecules of a protein called gp120. The virus gains entry to CD4 cells when gp120 grabs hold of CD4. However, it has been known since 1986 that binding of gp120 to CD4 alone is not sufficient to cause infection. If you try to infect mice with HIV, nothing happens, although mice do bear CD4 on their T helper cells. Researchers argued that a second 'handhold' or receptor on the CD4 cell was required. It was only in 1996 that the story of the elusive second receptor began to unravel.

Late in 1995, the veteran AIDS researcher Robert Gallo and his team showed that a group of chemical messengers called chemokines were able to suppress HIV infection. The strain of HIV in Gallo's experiments was called M-tropic, and is known to be involved in the early stages of infection. It is also the type most likely to be spread by sexual contact. M-tropic strains can affect macrophages, another type of white blood cell, as well as the CD4 cell – hence their name. Macrophages, by the way, are responsible for gobbling up and disposing of debris from dead cells, and they also engulf bacteria and other invading microbes. There is another strain of HIV called T-tropic, which tends to prefer infecting T helper cells, and emerges at later stages of infection. In contrast to M-tropic HIV, the T-tropic strains are spread chiefly by contaminated blood – that is, by injected drug use or by contaminated transfusion.

The trio of chemokines involved in Gallo's experiments were called RANTES, MIP-1α and MIP-1β. These molecules can suppress infection, but it is important to realise that there are other chemokines that have the opposite effect. Next, researchers from the US National Institute of Health announced the discovery of the second receptor, a protein called CXCR-4 which sits alongside CD4 and provides the essential helping hand to allow T-tropic strains of HIV into the cell. The following month, five different groups homed in on another second receptor, called CC CKR5, which is required for M-tropic virus infection. In subsequent weeks, the link between the chemokines and the second receptors was uncovered. Both second receptors bind to the chemokines. So the chemokines lock out HIV – both M and T tropic strains – by occupying that vital second receptor.

Meanwhile, powerful back-up evidence for the second receptor story was pouring in from human clinical studies. It has long been known that some people are naturally resistant to HIV, despite repeated exposure. There are haemophiliacs who have had repeated doses of contaminated blood products – and their partners, African prostitutes not using condoms, and homosexuals who admit to multiple partners whose HIV status is, at best, unknown. In April 1996, a team from the prestigious Aaron Diamond AIDS Research Centre in New York showed that the CD4 cells of a group of high-risk HIV negative volunteers were resistant to infection by the virus, at least in the test tube. Soon after, they homed in on two high-risk individuals and showed they had mutations in the gene that makes CC CKR5. The mutation meant that there was none of the second receptor on the surface of the CD4 cells of these people – so HIV was effectively locked out.

These observations were backed by population studies from the US and Belgium. We all have two copies of the CC CKR5 gene. In over 2000 people who were HIV positive, not one with two mutant copies of CC CKR5 was discovered. Furthermore, the incidence of people with one mutant copy was higher, at 16.2 per cent, in HIV negative controls than in the HIV positive group, where the corresponding figure was 10.8 per cent. This strongly suggests that mutation of the CC CKR5 gene does provide some protection against infection – at least from the M-tropic strain of HIV. There are also intriguing national differences in the incidence of the mutation; one per cent of Western Europeans have a double mutation, while 20 per cent have the single mutation. But no Africans or Asians appear to carry the CC CKR5 mutation.

Leading AIDS researchers have been quick to point out that these new insights provide an obvious lead for new drugs and vaccines. The impact that the second receptor story made was recorded by the journal *Science*, which has a watching brief over the status of scientific discoveries. Second receptors and protease inhibitors (also discussed later) got the joint award of the *Science* Breakthrough of the Year.

Now we know far more about how HIV enters CD4 cells. And once the CD4 cells are infected with HIV a number of symptoms such as weight loss and fever may occur. Within a few months of infection, antibodies to HIV appear in the blood and form the basis of a diagnostic test. So-called full-blown AIDS may take several years to develop after the original infection. Opportunistic infections usually set in when the CD4 count falls below 400 per cubic millimetre (the normal level is 1000 and it declines by 40 to 80 cells per cubic millimetre per annum after HIV infection). TB and pneumonia caused by the protozoan *Pneumocystis carinii* are common respiratory complications of AIDS. The central nervous system is another target, with dementias and various infections being common. Finally cancers such as lymphoma and, as previously mentioned, Kaposi's sarcoma are frequent occurrences in AIDS.

Viruses and chronic diseases It is becoming increasingly apparent that viruses, like bacteria, may play a role in chronic disease. In particular, there appears to be a link between viruses and cancer. The Epstein-Barr virus (EBV) is one of the best-studied cancer viruses; it is known to cause nasopharyngeal cancer which starts in the upper throat, behind the nose, and spreads through the nose and down to the neck. Nasopharyngeal cancer is rare in the West, but fairly common in the Far East. EBV also causes Burkitt's lymphoma, a tumour of the jaw and abdomen found in African children.

The virus that causes hepatitis B predisposes its victims to liver cancer, the commonest form of cancer in the world (although it is comparatively rare in the West). In the Far East 90 per cent of patients with a liver cancer have evidence of earlier hepatitis B infection. More recently it has been discovered that infection with the human papilloma virus (HPV) or the herpes simplex virus is strongly associated with cervical cancer. The infections initially cause genital warts or ulcers, and are both acquired by sexual intercourse with an infected person. Women who are infected should undergo cervical screening yearly (instead of every three years, which is the usual recommendation) to detect any pre-cancerous changes in the cells of the cervix.

Viruses have also been implicated in the development of a number of poorly understood conditions such as chronic fatigue syndrome (formerly known as myalgic encephalomyelitis or ME), rheumatoid arthritis and multiple sclerosis. There is also recent evidence that cytomegalovirus (CMV) infection may play a role in the development of coronary artery disease. And bornavirus infection, which affects both mammals and birds, may be linked with the development of both schizophrenia and clinical depression. Studies carried out in Japan and Germany showed that patients with these illnesses were up to six times more likely to have bornavirus infection than the general population.

It is becoming easier to detect viruses within human tissue samples by the use of probes for their DNA or RNA; such testing will eventually allow researchers to explore the links between viral infection and chronic disease more fully. And that will open up new treatment options such as vaccination.

The antibiotic revolution

At the beginning of this century people had good reason to fear infectious diseases – for there were no effective treatments. It was not uncommon for a woman to die of infection after childbirth. Look back in your own family history, and it is likely your great-grandparents lost one or more children to whooping cough, scarlet fever or diphtheria. Pneumonia too, could be a death sentence, and practically everyone harboured a secret fear of contracting sexually transmitted diseases, such as gonorrhoea or syphilis.

Then Paul Ehrlich's theory of the magic bullet – which was discussed in the previous chapter – was put to work. He was interested in chemicals that would kill microbes while leaving their human host alone, having noticed that some synthetic dyes are absorbed preferentially by parasites in human tissue. Ehrlich's antimicrobial bullet, however, turned out not to be a dye – but a compound containing arsenic. Scientists at the Liverpool School of Tropical Medicine had shown in 1905 that arsenic compounds (arsenicals) could protect mice from infection by parasites known as trypanosomes. Arsenicals are very toxic, but Ehrlich was determined to find one which would kill trypanosomes and other microbes while sparing the victim from side effects. The 606th arsenical he tested became the drug Salvarsan, which was used to kill the spirochaete bacteria that cause syphilis. Salvarsan – the first effective antibacterial compound – came onto the market in 1910.

Meanwhile the German biochemist Gerhard Domagk (1895–1964) began testing new dyes from the company I.G. Farben against streptococcal infection in mice. In 1932, he discovered that one dye, Prontosil Red, was particularly effective. One of the early volunteers in clinical trials of the dye was Domagk's own daughter who was seriously ill with sepsis contracted from a needle prick. The girl made a dramatic recovery, and Domagk was awarded a Nobel Prize for his work in 1939. It turned out – from later research in France – that Prontosil Red itself was not the active compound.

It is actually a prodrug – a compound which is inactive itself, but is converted into an active drug by the liver. Prontosil Red is converted into two compounds, one of which is sulphanilamide, a colourless molecule which kills the bacteria. Sulphanilamide, and related 'sulpha' drugs, are still used today in the treatment of urinary, sinus and ear infections.

These synthetic drugs are not, strictly speaking, antibiotics. This term is reserved for compounds like penicillin or erythromycin which come from bacteria or fungi and have antimicrobial activity. However, most doctors these days tend to call all anti-bacterial and anti-fungal drugs antibiotics (anti-viral drugs are not antibiotics in either sense of the word).

Bacteria and fungi produce antibiotics as a survival tactic. Species that could make a defensive compound which would kill their competitors, while they themselves remained unharmed, had an obvious advantage. In the last 60 years, this ancient form of chemical warfare has been harnessed for the benefit of humans and has saved millions of lives. The first success of the antibiotic revolution was, of course, penicillin.

In 1928 Scottish bacteriologist Alexander Fleming (1881–1955) left a Petri dish containing a culture of Staphylococcus open to the atmosphere while he went on holiday. On return, he noted that the plate had become contaminated – with the fungus *Penicillium notatum* – and part of the bacterial colony had been wiped out. He reasoned that the fungus must be producing some substance which was capable of killing bacteria.

Although Fleming had just stumbled on the first general-purpose antibiotic, he soon lost interest in his 'mould juice' because it was so hard to extract the penicillin from it. For many years, he doubted the drug would ever be used to treat infectious disease. He was to be proved wrong.

Penicillin was taken up again by Howard Florey and Ernst Chain of the Sir William Dunn School of Pathology in Oxford. Their work began in earnest in 1939, just as wartime conditions were beginning to make research especially difficult. Norman Heatley, their co-worker, recalls the makeshift equipment – trays, baths and biscuit tins – which was used to grow the mould so that enough penicillin could be extracted from it to treat a patient.

In February 1941, a 43-year-old policeman became the first person ever to receive penicillin. A sore on his mouth had become infected and dangerous abscesses developed around his eyes, face, and in his lungs. All other treatments had failed and he was desperately ill. Penicillin injections cleared the infection within days – but the drug was in such short supply that Florey and his team had to collect it from the patient's urine to recycle it. Soon supplies were exhausted. The infection returned with a vengeance, and the patient died just ten days after his astounding recovery.

This sad case was followed by better results. Several patients – including young children – made full recoveries from life-threatening infections after penicillin treatment. Even more significant were tests carried out at the Scottish Military Hospital in Egypt on wounded men in the desert army and at the Burns Unit in Oxford. Later on, Florey himself went out to North Africa, where he supervised the first major application of penicillin to war wounds. Convinced of penicillin's value to the war effort, the Oxford team approached the Ministry of Supply to discuss how production could be scaled up. The General Penicillin Committee was formed to oversee a highly confidential British-US drive to make enough penicillin to meet the needs of Allied troops.

Soon penicillin was being produced in secret all over the country – especially in and around London. Glaxo (now Glaxo Wellcome) of Greenford set up its first penicillin plant in a disused cheese factory in Aylesbury. This was followed by another in the top floor of a rubber factory in Watford, and a third in a converted cattle food factory in Stratford. Another key player in the penicillin drama, Kemball, Bishop and Co., used the basement of their Bromley-by-Bow premises, working on while incendiary bombs fell on the factory roof.

Penicillin-producing mould was grown in trays or in flasks known as 'bedpans' stacked up in their thousands wherever room could be found. The Americans grew their mould in giant fermenting vessels, but Britain stuck with the 'low-tech' method that had worked for Florey's team in the Oxford labs.

Worse than the bombing was the constant threat of contamination from airborne bugs. Some of these produce an enzyme which destroys penicillin. Exposure could destroy a whole batch of the precious drug. So everything and everyone which came into contact with the fermentation had to be spotlessly clean – no easy task under wartime conditions.

Like all living things, the mould needed food and it was fed a cheap diet of agricultural waste known as corn steep liquor. This had to be steam-sterilised before a team of 'penicillin girls' inoculated a tray or flask with a vessel containing the liquor. Once enough mould had grown on the surface of these vessels, it had to be harvested. Then the penicillin was extracted, dried and packed.

Labour was scarce, and of course penicillin production required new skills. But morale was high. Posters on the wall and pamphlets slipped into pay packets reminded workers how penicillin could save a loved one at the front.

One employee of Glaxo in Watford writing in the staff bulletin in 1946 wrote:

> D-day was not yet, and V-E day was a hope. Penicillin was wanted. We worked six days and five nights a week. We smelt of corn steep liquor. We cut our hands on broken flasks. We gave up our Bank Holidays. We cursed infection, but our output went up until at one time Glaxo in Watford was producing about 90% of all the penicillin made in this country.

It is a tribute to these men and women that by the time of the Sicily invasion campaign in 1943 the British pharmaceutical industry was producing enough penicillin for British troops – barely two years after supplies had run out while treating the first patient. And it must have been a great source of satisfaction to realise that thousands of lives – and limbs – were saved by penicillin in Europe and in Burma.

Penicillin first went on sale to the general public – as a prescription only drug – on June 1 1946. It is hard to overestimate the impact it had on public health. It undoubtedly played a major role in raising life expectancy. Penicillin even became the subject of a thriller. In *The Third Man* written by Graham Greene, a Berlin crime ring makes money by selling glucose as penicillin (they are both white powders).

The development of penicillin was rapidly followed by the discovery of the cephalosporin antibiotics. These come from the fungus *Cephalosporium* which was discovered among the microbial flora of sewage outflow by Guiseppe Brotzu of the University of Caligari, Sardinia.

But it was the Ukrainian émigré Selman Waksman (1888–1973) who tapped the biggest source of antibiotics. Soil contains around a billion microbes per cubic centimetre. Waksman argued that soil must be loaded with antibiotics that kept the microbial population under control. Otherwise the whole Earth would be overrun with bacteria and fungi. He began a big survey of antibiotic production in *Streptomyces* – a bacterial genus which is particularly abundant in the soil. His biggest success was the discovery of streptomycin from *S. griseus* which was developed into a drug for treating TB.

Most antibiotics kill bacteria, but some target fungi. One of the most important is nystatin, which was discovered by Elizabeth Hazen and Rachel Brown in 1949. Nystatin is named after the laboratories where it was discovered – the New York State Department of Health. By the mid-1950s, most of today's antibiotics had already been discovered. There are currently around 100 on the market.

Antibiotics act as molecular weapons

A good antibiotic shows a high level of selective toxicity – that is, it kills, or at least stops the growth of, the infecting organism without harming the host. To do this, the antibiotic's target must be a molecule which the organism has, but the host does not.

Penicillins, cephalosporins, and vancomycin show good selective toxicity because their target is the bacterial cell wall. Human cells do not have walls. The bacterial cell wall consists of a mesh of long, stringy molecules called peptidoglycan. Penicillin blocks an enzyme called glycopeptide transpeptidase, which co-ordinates the forging of cross-links between adjacent peptidoglycan chains. Inactivation of this enzyme stops the wall forming and, unprotected by this essential barrier between them and the environment, the bacteria 'burst'. This mechanism was not discovered until 1965 (years after penicillin had been introduced for general use).

Many other antibiotics act by inhibiting bacterial protein synthesis. This is not quite so specific – all living things must synthesise proteins, and the biochemical mechanisms by which they do so are remarkably similar. But at least bacteria use their own specific enzymes and other biochemical machinery to do so.

Protein synthesis is a complicated business (Figs 3.1 and 3.2). It is a two stage process which involves copying the 'message' in the DNA of a cell and then 'translating' it into a protein molecule. The message is 'written' in a chemical code which consists of four 'letters' – A, T, C and G. These stand for the four bases – small nitrogen-containing compounds – which are a key component of the DNA molecule, and are strung together along its length, like beads on a necklace. Groups of three bases make up 'words' known as codons. Each codon codes for an amino acid, so the whole message specifies the amino acid sequence of a protein. The message is 'copied' in the form of RNA – a chemical which is similar to DNA (Fig. 3.1). The DNA stays in the nucleus of a cell, but the messenger RNA (mRNA) can move into the cytoplasm to the site of protein synthesis (there are more details of about DNA and how it works in Chapter 11). Rifampicin, an anti-TB drug, and actinomycin work at this stage – which is known as transcription – by

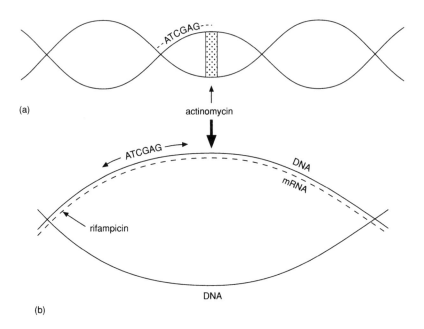

(a)   actinomycin

(b)

Fig. 3.1. How antibiotics inhibit transcription. Transcription is the first stage of protein synthesis. The DNA molecule is a double stranded helix (a) which must open up for the chemical code it carries to be copied. A small segment of coding 'ATCGAG' is shown. Actinomycin, shown as a shaded rectangle, binds to the double strand of DNA, preventing it from opening up so that transcription cannot occur. In (b), messenger RNA, represented by the broken line, has copied the message but the chemical bond between the first two letters of the message cannot be made in the presence of rifampicin, so the mRNA molecule is fatally flawed.

stopping the synthesis of bacterial mRNA. Actinomycin is so good at doing this that it is too toxic to be used as an antibiotic in humans; instead it is used in research, and as an anti-cancer drug.

Then the mRNA message passes to a molecular 'machine' called a ribosome. This consists of a large and small subunit, made of protein and a second form of RNA. The overall shape resembles that of a cottage loaf (Fig. 3.2). Of course, humans have ribosomes too; protein synthesis is an essential activity for all living cells and occurs by roughly the same mechanism in every organism. But bacterial and human ribosomes are sufficiently different for these antibiotics to show a good degree of selective toxicity. Tetracycline, streptomycin, chloramphenicol – a toxic antibiotic which is

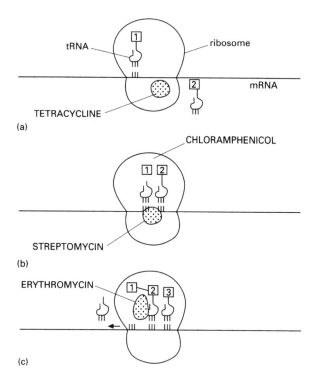

Fig. 3.2. How antibiotics block translation. The mRNA molecule runs through the two units of the ribosome like a tape through a tape head, and is 'read' in segments of three letters at a time (only one codon shown here). Successful protein synthesis depends upon the 'adaptor' molecule, tRNA, contacting the codon. In (a) the first tRNA has moved into place, carrying amino acid 1, but the approach of the second is blocked by a tetracycline molecule binding to the ribosome. In (b) amino acids 1 and 2, carried by adjacent tRNAs on the mRNA join to form the first link in the protein chain. The enzyme which creates this bond (not shown) is inhibited by chloramphenicol. Streptomycin binds the ribosome and jams the mRNA so the message is read incorrectly. Once two amino acids have joined together, they should move off the ribosome to allow the rest of the message to be read as shown in (c). Erythromycin blocks this movement by binding to the larger subunit of the ribosome.

only used as a last resort for life-threatening infection – and erythromycin all interfere with protein synthesis.

The mRNA message is held between the two subunits, which 'read' it like a tape (further details in Chapter 11). Each codon attracts its own amino acid, which is carried to the ribosome by an 'adaptor' molecule. This is yet another form of RNA, called transfer RNA (tRNA) which has a triplet of bases called an anticodon at one end, and the amino acid at the other end. The anticodon recognises the appropriate codon and so moves into position with its amino acid. Tetracycline acts by binding to the small subunit of the bacterial ribosome and blocking the approach of tRNA.

Streptomycin also binds to the small subunit. It causes the mRNA message to become misaligned in the tape reader, so that the codon is read wrongly. Proteins are still made, but they are completely non-functional because their amino acid sequences are wrong.

Once an amino acid is in position, it has to be bolted onto the rest of the growing protein chain via an enzyme called peptidyl transferase. Chloramphenicol inhibits this enzyme, so the protein chain terminates prematurely. Finally, once an amino acid has been attached to the protein chain, it needs to move along so that the next amino acid with its anticodon can move into position. Erythromycin binds to the large subunit and blocks this translocation, so that the new protein chain gets stuck on the ribosome.

All cells contain DNA as a double helical molecule which must unwind, separate, and replicate into two new DNA molecules each time the cell divides to make two new cells. Bacteria reproduce by this kind of cell division. The quinolone antimicrobial drugs such as ciprofloxacin, which is used to treat gut infections, inhibit DNA gyrase, the enzyme that helps the new DNA molecule separate from its parent molecule. Under attack from a quinolone, bacteria cannot divide.

The sulpha drugs act as anti-metabolites. That is, they stand in for a vital chemical that the bacteria need – in this case para-aminobenzoic acid (PABA). Bugs need PABA to assemble folic acid, a vital ingredient in the synthesis of the building blocks of DNA and RNA. As humans get folic acid ready-made from their diet (we do not have the molecular machinery to make it ourselves), the folic acid anti-metabolites should not affect us and are therefore a good example of selective toxicity. A related drug is trimethoprim, an inhibitor of the enzyme dihydrofolate reductase (DHFR), which acts on folic acid itself. Humans have their own DHFR enzyme, but the affinity of trimethoprim for bacterial DHFR is 50,000 times greater than its affinity for the human version.

The problem of antibiotic resistance

Microbes, and bacteria in particular, are a moving target as far as drug therapy is concerned. Like all living things, microbes are continually evolving. As mentioned above, the bacteria that existed on Earth over three billion years ago were already guarding their resources and territory with a sophisticated arsenal of antibiotic weapons. Naturally, the species under attack evolved defences against the antibiotics which were being trained on them; this is the basis of today's clinical problem of antibiotic resistance – the existence of microbes which are no longer sensitive to the drugs used to treat them. Incidentally, resistance can develop to synthetic antimicrobials, as well as to antibiotics. Here we will use the term antibiotic resistance to refer to the clinical problem affecting *both types* of antimicrobial drug.

The problems of antibiotic resistance became apparent within a few years of the introduction of antibiotic therapy. In 1941, fewer than one per cent of *Staphylococcus aureus* strains were resistant to the newly introduced penicillin (a strain is a group within a species of bacteria that differs only slightly from other strains of that species, and normally arises from a single bacterial colony). By 1946, 14 per cent of *S. aureus* strains were resistant and by 1948 38 per cent. Today fewer than 1 per cent of all strains of this species – which is responsible for pimples, boils, food poisoning and respiratory infections – are sensitive to penicillin.

The scale of the problem The problem of antibiotic resistance exists both in hospitals and, increasingly, in the community. There is little doubt that people are now dying of hospital infections who would have survived five or ten years ago. There are strains of *Enterococcus* – a gut bacterium that normally causes few problems – which are causing untreatable infections in renal and intensive care units. They are untreatable because they have become resistant to all known antibiotics, as have strains of *Pseudomonas* which are turning up in patients with cystic fibrosis, causing potentially fatal respiratory infections.

Another serious problem is the emergence of methicillin resistant *Staphylococcus aureus* (MRSA). This organism is now said to affect over half of all hospitals in the UK. It is resistant not just to methicillin, but to many other antibiotics. Doctors often have to resort to vancomycin – often called the antibiotic of 'last resort' – in MRSA. Vancomycin would not usually be the first choice – it is expensive and has to be given by injection. It can be toxic to the ears and kidneys, and sometimes causes flushing, chills and fever, as well as inflammation at the site of injection.

Until recently antibiotic resistant microbes were found mainly in hospitals. Now they are moving out into the community. The most common is perhaps *Streptococcus pneumoniae*, which is responsible for pneumonia and ear infections. This is on the increase and some strains are resistant to all antibiotics but vancomycin and cephalosporins. There are also resistant strains of *Haemophilus influenzae*, the cause of a life-threatening form of meningitis, on the loose. And recently, a strain of *Salmonella typhimurium* resistant to all known antibiotics emerged. Cases of food poisoning related to this particular bacterium have tripled in Britain over the last few years. Because the bug is resistant to treatment the infection is said to be ten times more deadly than normal food poisoning.

On a global scale drug resistant TB is a growing problem. It occurs mainly in AIDS patients and currently South Africa is the country most affected, with around four per cent of all cases being drug resistant. But there have also been outbreaks in other major cities such as New York and London.

How bacteria become resistant to antimicrobial drugs Resistance to antibiotics occurs in three main ways. First, the bacterium may break down the antibiotic. This is the main mechanism of resistance to penicillins and cephalosporins. They contain a characteristic chemical group called the beta lactam ring. This is easily broken down by enzymes called beta lactamases which are produced by many bacteria.

Secondly, the resistant microbes can stop the antibiotic from getting inside their cells, or can even pump it out once it is inside. So-called gram negative bacteria have pores inside their cell walls through which the antibiotic molecules can travel. Loss or narrowing of these channels means that the antibiotic can no longer get inside. This mechanism has caused the emergence of resistant *Pseudomonas aeruginosa* in hospitals.

Finally, the molecular target of the antibiotic can change. When the structure of the enzyme DHFR alters its shape, for instance, the affinity of trimethoprim for it decreases – leading to the development of trimethoprim resistance.

All these evolutionary changes start off as changes in the genes of the microbes. These get translated into changes within the microbial cell, such as a subtle alteration in the shape of an enzyme. These genetic changes may occur by simple mutation. Each time a bacterium splits into two its DNA is copied and mistakes – known as mutations – may happen which change the coded message for an enzyme. More often though, complete genes are transferred between bacterial species by bacterial 'sex'. Antibiotic resistance genes are carried on tiny circles of DNA called plasmids. Two bacteria can join up by a tube in a process called conjugation, and the plasmid can pass from one to another through the tube.

Normally, having antibiotic resistance would not be to the benefit of an organism. In fact until recently it was thought that it might decrease the fitness of the microbe. However, recent experiments by researchers at Emory University in Atlanta, suggest that the bacteria evolve further compensating mutations which increase their fitness.

Use of antibiotics is a selective pressure favouring resistant microbes. It works like this. Supposing you take a course of ampicillin for a throat infection. You start off with a normal population of, say, *Staphylococcus aureus* in your throat. Inevitably some of the microbes will be more resistant to the ampicillin than others. The more sensitive ones will be killed within the first couple of days of ampicillin treatment, and the population then in your throat will be relatively more resistant to the drug. Suppose you then feel better and forget to take the rest of the course – which would have been needed to kill off the resistant bugs in the population. You have now shifted the balance in favour of resistant bacteria. Next time you have a throat infection expect it to be harder to cure, because you did not complete the course the first time. The problem of not completing courses of antibiotics is particularly prevalent in the treatment of TB where sufferers may be homeless and not under medical supervision. Courses of treatment for TB can be very long – up to a year in some cases.

Then again, some people give antibiotics to their friends and family, while in some countries they are even available over the counter for unsupervised use. Doctors are sometimes at fault. According to a report in The Lancet in 1996, up to 40 per cent of patients visiting their GP with a 'cold' get antibiotics. A cold is a viral infection and viruses are not killed by antibiotics. In a minority of colds – say one in five – there is a co-existing bacterial infection in the upper respiratory tract and this may respond to the antibiotic. But, given time, the immune system would probably throw off both infections. Prescription of an antibiotic for a cold is usually unnecessary, and in the long term actually harmful – for it encourages the emergence of resistant bacteria. So why do doctors do it? Probably because they feel under pressure to 'do something' for their patient.

Doctors also over-use the broad spectrum antibiotics which attack a wide range of bacteria; they tend to prescribe them while waiting for laboratory tests to confirm which organism is responsible for the infection. It might be wiser to wait, and then prescribe something more specific which will exert selective pressure on fewer species than a broad spectrum drug. The damage that can be done by over-frequent antibiotic prescribing is illustrated by a recent report on meningitis clusters. Towns in the UK which had up to nine times more cases of meningitis than average had 50 per cent more antibiotic prescriptions, particularly for erythromycin.

The widespread use of antibiotics as a prophylactic in agriculture creates a selective pressure on resistant microbes just as their clinical use in humans does. Resistant bacteria start to turn up in poultry, beef and lamb which are then consumed by the fast food market. There is a particular problem with the veterinary antibiotic avoparcin, because it resembles vancomycin. Once a bacterium is resistant to avoparcin, it is likely to be resistant to vancomycin too. In fact vancomycin resistant Enterococci have already been found in meat and meat products in Germany, although not in meat from organic farms that did not use antibiotics. Ideally, antibiotics that resemble those used in humans would not be used at all. Germany and Denmark have already banned avoparcin; now the European Union has recommended a continent-wide ban.

Antibiotic resistance has the potential to become a major public health emergency within the next few years; but it need not be. Many simple measures could be put in place. First, we could try harder to limit the spread of infection. The public and medical profession alike have become complacent. Simple hygiene measures, such as hand washing before meals, have been abandoned. People do not worry about sending children to school with infections, and struggle into work themselves when they are ill – infecting their colleagues. Vaccination is no longer routine in some parts of the UK. And fit healthy people still expect antibiotics for infections, rather than resting and relying on their immune system to deal with the problem.

As far as antibiotic treatments are concerned, there is much to be said for keeping some drugs in reserve, or monitoring their consumption. And anything that can be done to widen the antibiotic armoury will be especially valuable. The signs are that some drug companies are now awakening to this challenge.

Variations on the themes of existing antibiotics have been successful. For instance imipenem is a penicillin where access to the beta lactam ring is restricted by chemical modification, so bacterial enzymes cannot break it down. Another way of reviving the fortunes of antibiotics which have been rendered useless by resistance is to pair them with a second compound which tackles the resistance mechanism. Augmentin is one of many examples of this strategy; it consists of the antibiotic amoxycillin and clavulanic acid. On its own the beta lactam ring of amoxycillin would easily be broken down by the beta lactamase enzymes of resistant bacteria. But clavulanic acid, which is not an antibiotic in its own right, also has a beta lactam ring and can bind more tightly to beta lactamase than the corresponding ring in amoxycillin. So clavulanic acid effectively disarms the beta lactamase, leaving the amoxycillin to go in for the kill.

Many companies are searching for novel sources of new antibiotics. There are compounds under development which have come from moths, beetles, sharks, cow saliva, and frogs. Many of these are so-called host defence peptides; they work in a completely different way from conventional antibiotics, by punching holes in bacterial cell walls. And there are still many new antibiotics to be discovered in microbes themselves. Scientists at Heriot-Watt University have discovered that bacteria that live on seaweed make compounds that can defeat MRSA.

It may also be possible to revive an idea from the pre-antibiotic era, based on using the natural enemies of bacteria as a means of attack. Bacteriophage are viruses that prey on bacteria. Each phage is specific to one bacterial species, and they do not attack humans. Experiments done on phage therapy in the 1930s were promising but lacked rigour. The idea has been taken up again by Jim Bull of the University of Texas and Bruce Levin of Emory University in Atlanta. They have treated mice infected with *E. coli* with phage and found it to be more effective than standard antibiotic treatment. In fact phage therapy has been practised for many years in Georgia in the former Soviet Union, although the work is little known in the West. In the Georgian State Paediatric Hospital, phage treatment is used for a wide range of infections.

Finding new microbial targets to attack is an important strategy, although limited by the relative simplicity of a microbe's biochemistry (at least compared to that of a human). Researchers at pharmaceutical giant Merck recently reported on a new compound which attacks the mechanism by which some bacteria make their toxins. Another company, Pharmacia and Upjohn, has a new group of antibiotics called the oxazolidinones in late clinical development. These inhibit the initiation of mRNA translation (Fig. 3.2) and show excellent activity against MRSA, vancomycin resistant enterococci and drug resistant TB. Two of these antibiotics, eperezolid and linezolid, could reach the market in the next year or so.

Genetic studies are bound to reveal many new targets for potential antibiotic therapy. The complete genomes of a number of pathogenic bacteria have already been mapped or are being mapped (see also Chapter 11). Glaxo Wellcome, the company which did so much to make penicillin widely available, has developed a new gene-based strategy called IVET, which is short for *in vitro* expression technology. It is known that bacteria express genes during infection that they do not express under other circumstances. The aim is to identify these and their products to provide new targets for antibiotics.

Antimalarial drugs

Like antibiotics, antimalarial drugs are beginning to lose their power to fight infection because of the increasing problem of resistance. The three front line drugs in the treatment of malaria are chloroquine, quinine, and mefloquine. These clear the malaria parasites from the blood within 24 hours, although their mechanism of action remains unclear. Chloroquine has few serious side effects but *Plasmodium falciparum*, which accounts for around half of all cases of malaria, is resistant to it in most parts of the world where the disease is endemic (including Africa, the Middle East and Latin America). The drug does not appear able to enter resistant parasites. Quinine (whose use dates back to the 17th century) and mefloquine are more toxic drugs, but are still effective in treating malaria caused by chloroquine resistant strains.

Pyrimethamine and proguanil are slower acting drugs which also eliminate the parasites from the blood. Like trimethoprim, which was discussed earlier, they act as folic acid antimetabolites, inhibiting the enzyme DHFR. They are selectively toxic to the parasites because they have 1000 times the affinity for parasite DHFR when compared to the corresponding human enzyme. Sometimes they are combined with a sulphonamide which, as mentioned earlier, knocks out an earlier step in the purine and pyrimidine nucleic acid building blocks.

Malaria caused by *P. vivax* and the rare *P. ovale* may flare up again, even after successful treatment, because the parasites lie dormant in the liver. The drug primaquine, whose exact mode of action is not well understood, can eradicate the liver infection – but is quite toxic and is generally used once the parasites have first been eliminated from the blood by chloroquine or a related drug.

Prophylaxis against malaria by taking one or more of the above drugs – except quinine, which is too toxic for long-term use – is usually recommended for anyone visiting areas where malaria is endemic. The expansion in business and leisure travel to tropical countries has put increasing numbers of people from the United States and Europe at risk of contracting malaria. Prophylactic drugs should be taken for one or two weeks before departure, and then for a full four weeks after return. Failure to follow this programme is a major factor in the 2000 or so cases of malaria (some of them fatal) which occur in Britain each year on return from a malarious area.

Travellers are usually prescribed either chloroquine and proguanil, or mefloquine (Lariam), a newer drug. Mefloquine is associated with serious neuropsychiatric side effects such as psychosis, epileptic fits, and mood swings. According to a recent report in the British Medical Journal, these affected one person in 140 taking Lariam – about eight times more than those taking the older drugs. And up to 40 per cent of people taking any of the prophylactics suffered some side effects, although most of these were fairly minor. The report concluded that mefloquine should only be taken if travelling to a high risk area or if chloroquine resistance was widespread. But the net effect of the adverse publicity has been that some people are taking the distinctly risky option of travelling without taking any prophylaxis.

There is an urgent need for new drugs against malaria, given the spread of resistance against the few in the current portfolio and the problem of side effects with propylactics. So the emergence of artemether, an antimalarial which comes from the sweet wormwood plant, *Artemesia annua*, is especially welcome. Artemether is the active ingredient of qinghaosu, a traditional Chinese remedy for fever. It clears *P. falciparum* from the blood and in clinical trials it worked as well as quinine in the treatment of severe malaria. Overall mortality was the same in both groups of patients, but artemether acted more quickly. It also has the advantage that it can be given orally, whereas quinine has to be delivered via intravenous injection.

There are a number of other potential compounds that could be developed as antimalarials. The problem is that few drug companies appear to be prepared to take them on, probably because the people most affected by malaria may be unable to purchase even the cheapest of any new drugs. Many researchers and policy experts are now calling for the industry to 'ringfence' funds for malaria, and to enter into collaborations with governments to find ways of addressing this global problem.

Meanwhile, low-tech approaches can give good results. The use of insecticide impregnated bed nets in the Gambia and Kenya has dramatically cut childhood mortality from malaria.

Antiviral drugs

It is difficult to treat viral infections with drugs. The virus is a parasite inside the host cell, hijacking its biochemical machinery which then becomes inextricably tangled with its own. So it is hard to hit the virus selectively without damaging the host cell. Viral diseases are best treated by preventative measures; that means vaccination, which is discussed in the next section.

However, a few effective antiviral drugs have been developed. The most successful of these is acyclovir which is used to treat *Herpes simplex* and *Varicella zoster* infections. *H. simplex* causes cold sores and genital herpes, while *V. zoster* causes chicken pox and shingles, both potentially dangerous infections in people with reduced immunity. Acyclovir is selective for its viral target in two ways. First, it is a prodrug which is activated by viral enzymes – but hardly at all by the equivalent human enzyme. And second, it acts like one of the building blocks of DNA; *Herpes* viral DNA polymerase (the enzyme which assembles the DNA molecule from its building blocks) mistakenly binds to activated acyclovir molecules and is effectively inhibited. Human DNA polymerase does not bind the drug. However, acyclovir is not active against other viruses.

A new antiviral drug, from Glaxo Wellcome, which could be on the market in a year or so, is zanamivir which acts against both the A and B strains of influenza. The starting point for the rational design of zanamivir was the X-ray crystal structure of one of the influenza virus enzymes, neuraminidase. This helps spread infection by processing new viral particles so that they can escape from their host cells and invade other cells. By study of the active site of neuraminidase on a computer screen, scientists in Australia, and at Glaxo in the UK, were able to pick molecules which would block it from a computer library of chemical structures. In recent clinical trials zanamivir was tested as a nasal spray in healthy volunteers infected with influenza virus. When used before infection, as prophylaxis, zanamivir was able to protect the volunteers; only five per cent of them reported flu symptoms. When given after infection it reduced the length of the illness compared with volunteers who were on placebo; symptoms such as cough and sneezing cleared up rapidly, and laboratory tests showed a marked decrease in the number of viruses. Now there is a related drug, from Gilead Sciences of Foster City, California, which can be taken as a pill. If clinical trials work out, both drugs should be on the market before the year 2000.

The main stimulus for the development of new antiviral drugs has been the emergence of AIDS. Until recently, the only drug available was zidovudine (AZT). Like acyclovir, AZT is activated to create a mimic of a DNA building block, known as a nucleoside. It binds to reverse transcriptase, an enzyme which is essential to the reproduction of HIV. Unfortunately AZT alone is not very effective in reducing mortality from AIDS. It is also associated with side effects such as severe anaemia and neutropenia (a decrease in the number of white cells called neutrophils in the blood, which leads to increased susceptibility to infection). Worse, HIV has evolved resistance to AZT which greatly limits its effectiveness.

The next stage in treating HIV/AIDS was to use AZT in combination with a second nucleoside analogue – either ddI or ddC. This so-called combination therapy was more effective than AZT alone in slowing progression to AIDS. Then the HIV protease inhibitors were discovered (as discussed in the previous chapter). Trials, on both recently infected patients and patients with advanced AIDS, suggest that these new drugs are also best used in combination. Triple therapy – AZT, a second nucleoside analogue, and a protease inhibitor – is fast becoming the 'gold standard' of AIDS treatment.

Trials of triple therapy show it can effectively eliminate HIV from the blood for many months. This decrease in viral load can now be translated into increased survival times. One study showed that of people with fewer than 10,000 viral particles per ml of blood, 70 per cent survived for more than ten years, while only 30 per cent of patients with a higher load than this survived for the same length of time. The latest trial, carried out by Roche, involved the largest number of patients to date and shows a clear survival benefit with triple therapy. The details were as follows: 3485 patients were randomised to four treatment groups (note, there was no placebo group). They received AZT alone, saquinavir (Roche's protease inhibitor) plus AZT, AZT plus ddC, or triple therapy of AZT, ddC and saquinavir. Of the 125 deaths occurring in the 18 month period of the trial there were 39, 34, 31 and 21 respectively in each treatment group.

If a patient is given triple therapy early on in the course of infection, it may stop the virus from destroying his immune system. Each drug attacks the virus at different points in its life-cycle, so together they keep its multiplication rate low. This is important, because the less the virus multiplies the less chance it has to mutate and evolve resistance to the drugs.

The effects of triple therapy, where it has been used, have been amazing. Patients under threat of what they thought was a death sentence are now returning to work and making plans for the future. AIDS wards are being closed down and resources concentrated on outpatient support. HIV/AIDS is now being seen as a chronic disease, rather like diabetes or arthritis, which the patient must learn to live with.

The drawbacks of triple therapy are that it is very expensive (around

$15,000 a year to treat a single patient, which represents around 20 to 30 times the average income of an African patient). The treatment regime is complicated; some AIDS patients take up to 100 pills a day in all. It is also not known what the long-term side effects of protease inhibitors may be, because the drugs are so new. However, all three have significant interactions with other drugs – particularly with rifampicin, an anti-TB drug which many AIDS patients may find themselves taking.

And triple therapy is not really a 'cure' because the virus could still be lurking in the lymph glands or other body tissues. One patient who stopped taking the drug – after 78 weeks, when his blood and lymph were clear – was found to have high levels of HIV in his blood only a week later.

However, there is no doubt that HIV protease inhibitors have been the success story for the pharmaceutical industry of the 1990s. The HIV drug market was worth $1500 million in 1996 and this is set to double by the year 1998. The three drugs currently on the market, other than saquinavir (Invirase), are ritonavir (Norvir, from Abbott Laboratories), indinavir (Crixivan, Merck Sharp and Dohme) and nelfinavir (Viracept, Agouron). There are several other, possibly more potent, protease inhibitors in the pipeline.

Vaccines protect the body against infection

Many infections clear up without the aid of antimicrobial drugs thanks to the defensive actions of the body's immune system. If the same infection occurs again, the body will often be able to throw it off before it takes hold, because the immune system responds more quickly the second time round – as if the first occasion was a mere rehearsal, and the second the actual performance.

The aim of vaccination is to exploit this natural process. There are several types of vaccine; they all have the effect of simulating the disease to the extent of prompting an immune response. Once alerted, the immune system is ready to go when challenged by the real infection.

Edward Jenner (1749–1823) was the founding father of vaccination. In the 18th century people who had survived smallpox would bear marks (pocks) on their skin from the disease. Milkmaids were noted for their clear complexions suggesting that they rarely contracted smallpox. Jenner surmised that cowpox – a related but much milder disease which was contracted, as the name suggests, from cows – conferred immunity to smallpox.

Determined to test out this theory, he made a crude vaccine of cowpox virus taken from a milkmaid called Sarah Nelmes and, using a thorn as a syringe, injected it into eight-year-old James Phipps on 14 May 1796. A few weeks later he daringly injected the boy with smallpox. To everyone's relief the boy remained healthy. It is a fitting tribute to Jenner that less than two centuries later, smallpox was eradicated worldwide. Case tracing and quarantine played a major role in this medical triumph, but there is little doubt that large scale vaccination was also vital.

Jenner's achievement was all the more remarkable given that nothing was known, at the time, of microbes or the immune system. Little happened for nearly a century; then Louis Pasteur (1822–1895), who laid the foundations of microbiology, developed vaccines for anthrax and rabies. In 1921–1923, French bacteriologists Albert Calmette and Camille Guérin developed the BCG vaccine for TB, and around this time vaccines against diphtheria and tetanus were also discovered. Then, in the 1950s and 1960s, came vaccines against polio, measles and rubella. By this time, the complexities of the immune system and the mechanisms of disease were far better understood. But vaccines for other infectious diseases did not then follow automatically.

In fact all the easy vaccines have already been made. There are currently over 100 new vaccines in the pipeline; developing these has been far more of a challenge. Today there are several types of vaccine. Some are still based on Jenner's original principle – live virus, but of a weakened (known as attenuated) strain which cannot harm the recipient. Live viruses do carry a risk though – they could mutate into a pathogenic form. An example of one of the new live vaccines is one against cholera, in which the gene for cholera toxin has been removed by genetic engineering. An alternative is to use dead virus. These vaccines can generate an effective response, but again there are safety considerations; all the virus must be killed during manufacture.

A vaccine works by 'presenting' an antigen to the immune system. The antigen is one of the proteins which the infecting microbe carries on its surface, and it stimulates the immune system. The antigen produces antibodies which can either label the microbe for destruction by white blood cells which can engulf it, or cause its destruction in other ways. Once produced the antibodies will stay in the blood, usually for years.

So there is no reason why a vaccine should consist of the whole virus – the appropriate antigen should be enough, and safer too, as a protein molecule cannot set up an infection. Thanks to genetic engineering techniques purified antigens can now be made in quantity in fermenters. The first genetically engineered vaccine was for human hepatitis B. This is a severe, and potentially fatal, infection of the liver which greatly increases the chance of developing liver cancer. The vaccine is made by transferring the gene for a carefully selected antigen from the surface of the hepatitis B virus into yeast (for details see Chapter 11). The yeast multiply in the fermenter, creating large amounts of antigen as they do so.

It is not even the whole protein molecule which is required to stimulate immunity in most cases, but rather loops of amino acids on the surface of the protein called epitopes. These short strings of amino acids, known as peptides, are easily made by a machine called a peptide synthesiser. If epitopes can be identified by experiment, then peptide vaccines can be developed.

The immune system is divided into two parts. Humoral immunity involves the production of antibodies, while cell-mediated immunity involves the activation of white cells and production of certain chemicals known as cytokines. As understanding of the immune system has grown the idea of developing vaccines that stimulate cell-mediated immunity, rather than antibody production, has gained ground.

Cell-mediated immunity is stimulated when a virus gets inside a cell, hiding from antibodies. The infected cell sticks pieces of protein from the virus on its surface, signalling to the immune system to destroy it. These proteins are often those inside the virus rather than on its surface, and they tend to mutate less than surface proteins.

These considerations have led to the development of DNA vaccines. These are genes that code for these proteins and produce them inside cells so that the cell-mediated immunity can be stimulated. The first of these to be tested in animals was an influenza vaccine made of the gene that codes for one of the inner proteins. The success of this approach was demonstrated by the fact that the experimental mice were protected from strains of influenza from 1934 and 1968 – during which time period surface proteins, on which a traditional vaccine would have been based, would have mutated rapidly, while inner proteins had hardly altered. DNA vaccines for TB, hepatitis and a number of other diseases are being developed.

Undoubtedly the two main targets for vaccine development are AIDS and malaria. Indeed it is hard to see how these diseases can be controlled without a vaccine; the majority of people who suffer them cannot afford the drugs on offer, even if these were effective. For AIDS there are 20 vaccines in some kind of clinical trials, but only two – in Thailand – in phase III. There are perhaps 30 more at an earlier stage of development. Production of a successful vaccine has been hampered by several factors. First, the very nature of AIDS involves failure of the immune system; antibodies are produced but fail to clear the infection. In other diseases, the antibodies work so it is reasonable to try to produce them with a vaccine. So more basic research is needed to identify the correct immune response which a vaccine should elicit. Second, there is no good animal model to test the vaccine in. Chimpanzees can be infected with HIV, but they do not get AIDS. On the other hand, macaques do get AIDS, but on infection with simian immuno-deficiency virus (SIV) which is not HIV but is rather a monkey equivalent.

Malaria is a complex target for vaccine development because the infection goes through so many different stages as discussed earlier. A peptide vaccine has been developed by Colombian scientist Manuel Patarroyo, based on several different antigens. Patarroyo donated his work to the WHO; unfortunately, clinical trials have given conflicting results on efficacy. It cut the incidence of *P. falciparum* malaria by one- to two-thirds in trials in Latin America, and gave similar results in Tanzanian children. But trials in children in the Gambia and Thailand appeared to show no protective effects. However, further investigations are being carried out. Some researchers think the vaccine may be more effective if given to younger children. There are also three other malaria vaccines under development. One of these, from Australian scientists, is already undergoing clinical trials in Papua New Guinea.

So infection will continue to be a battleground fought out on the worldwide stage. Persuading the drug companies to fight their corner may be difficult, as some of the poorest people in the world are those who stand to benefit most.

Drugs against infection and vaccines have had a profound impact on people around the world in the past 50 years. The antibiotic revolution was to be followed by another pharmaceutical breakthrough – one which affected people's lives in quite a different way. The story of hormonal contraceptives and related drugs will be told in the next chapter.

4

The hormonal revolution

Hormones are among the most widely prescribed drugs in the world. Unlike antibiotics, they do not attack an invisible enemy. Instead, they intervene in the body's control systems. In the beginning, hormone medicines, like insulin, were used to treat diseases caused by a lack of one or other of the body's natural hormones. Since the 1960s, however, hormone drugs have revolutionised the lives of millions of women around the world by providing for the first time a reliable, long-term, method of contraception. And as these same women approach the menopause, they can now opt to take hormone replacement therapy – a choice which may have a dramatic impact on their health in later years.

The world around us is constantly changing. We tend to attach the most importance to social, political and cultural change, but our bodies have to cope with more basic environmental fluctuations in order to survive for 70 years or more. Enzymes, as we saw in Chapter 1, are the driving force behind the chemistry of life. To function, they need the right temperature, level of acidity, salt concentration, an adequate supply of raw materials and so on within the cells which are their workplace. The body needs to maintain this inner environment in the face of a whole range of outer stresses. Its remarkable ability to do so is known as homeostasis, and it all works through the endocrine system through the action of hormones.

The endocrine system consists of a number of glands (Fig. 4.1) which respond to biochemical signals – such as a fall in blood sugar – by synthesising and secreting tiny amounts of one, or more, hormones into the bloodstream. The biochemical signals themselves convey information from outside (low blood sugar means you missed breakfast, for example). The endocrine system organises the body's response to this message.

Hormones are chemical messengers. They link the endocrine glands with the other organs of the body. Once a hormone reaches its target, it alters the physiological activity of that cell or tissue. They are powerful chemicals;

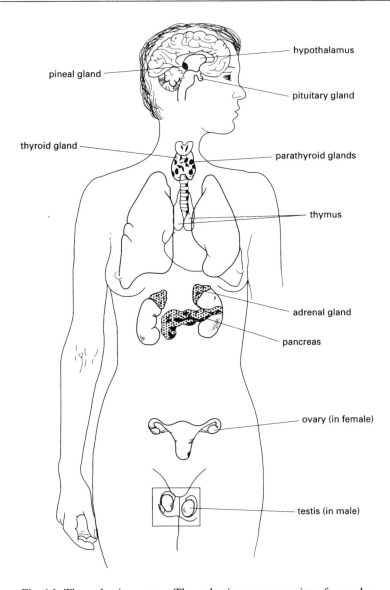

Fig. 4.1. The endocrine system. The endocrine system consists of a number of glands, each of which secretes one or more different hormones into the bloodstream. The hormones act upon specific target organs, giving rise to any cellular and physiological changes which are necessary to keep the body's inner environment stable.

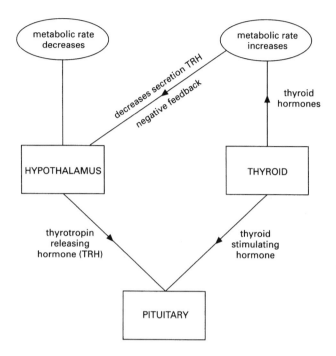

Fig. 4.2. How negative feedback works. Negative feedback is the basic mechanism of homeostasis. If metabolic rate falls, the hypothalamus responds by releasing thryrotropin releasing hormone which triggers the release of thyroid hormones via the action of the pituitary. Thyroid hormones act directly on cells, raising the metabolic rate. But this increase also has the effect of 'switching off' the hormonal chain of action which produced it. The net result is maintenance of a steady inner environment.

generally a tiny amount has a big effect, and they are only secreted when needed.

Control of hormone secretion (and therefore homeostasis) occurs by a negative feedback type of mechanism (Fig. 4.2). In negative feedback, any change in a system (in this case the body's internal chemistry is the system) produces a response that tends to restore the status quo. As an example, suppose the metabolic rate of the body – which, put simply, is the rate at which glucose fuel is being burned in cells – drops. To keep the body supplied with biochemical energy, it is desirable that the metabolic rate should be roughly constant. If it falls, something will have to happen to make it rise again.

The hypothalamus (Fig. 4.1) keeps a close watch on such matters, by responding to levels of body chemicals in the bloodstream. When it gets a signal that metabolic rate is falling, it pumps out thyrotropin-releasing hormone (TRH) which acts upon the nearby pituitary gland, nudging it into producing another hormone, thyroid stimulating hormone (TSH). As the name suggests, this acts in turn upon the thyroid gland which secretes thyroid hormones (known as thyroxine and triiodothyronine). The thyroid hormones act upon most cells in the body, causing them to speed up their metabolic rate. The emergency call picked up by the hypothalamus has been acted on, order has been restored – and all through a chain of hormonal messages. And should the metabolic rate start to overshoot the body's set-point, the feedback mechanism will work in the opposite direction – pulling in the various hormones, so that the metabolism can calm down a bit.

How hormones work on their targets

Hormones can be divided into two broad categories on the basis of their chemical structures. Those which are water-soluble, such as insulin, are mainly peptides, proteins or catecholamines (simple organic compounds containing nitrogen). The others are fat-soluble and include the thyroid hormones and steroid hormones. The steroids are a biologically diverse group including hormones (such as the sex hormones testosterone and oestrogen and the stress hormone cortisol), vitamin D, and cholesterol. All steroid molecules have a characteristic structure consisting of three six-membered and one five-membered ring of carbon atoms fused together.

The two classes of hormone interact differently with their targets. Water soluble hormones cannot pass inside the fatty membrane of the cell, so they have to exert their effects from outside. They do this by the so-called second messenger mechanism. First they dock onto a membrane-bound receptor protein (Fig. 4.3). The hormone–receptor complex activates a nearby protein in the membrane, called the G protein, which in turn activates a membrane-bound enzyme, adenylyl cyclase. This catalyses the conversion of an important molecule called adenosine triphosphate (ATP) into a cyclic molecule called cyclic AMP (cAMP). The hormone is known as the first messenger in this scheme, while cAMP is the second messenger. It is cAMP which produces the cellular response, by activating enzymes known as kinases. cAMP is known to increase production of energy in liver cells and

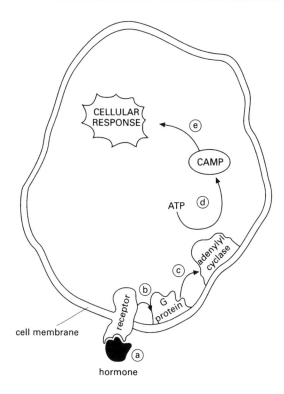

Fig. 4.3. How the second messenger mechanism of hormone action works. (a) A soluble hormone, such as insulin, binds to a receptor protein which spans the membrane. (b) The act of binding activates a nearby G-protein, bound to the inner surface of the membrane. (c) This in turn activates the enzyme adenylyl cyclase (d) and the enzyme converts ATP into cAMP, the second messenger. (e) cAMP orchestrates a number of cellular and physiological responses.

increase contraction of cardiac muscle, as well as producing many other responses.

Lipid-soluble hormones can get inside the cells, where they are involved in what is known as the direct gene mechanism (Fig. 4.4). The hormone binds to a receptor protein, and the hormone–receptor complex drifts towards the nucleus of the cell where it locks onto a specific sequence of DNA that is part of its control region. The net effect is of taking the brakes off the gene, so that it can turn on its protein synthesis machinery. Each gene makes its own individual protein. So the physiological response to the

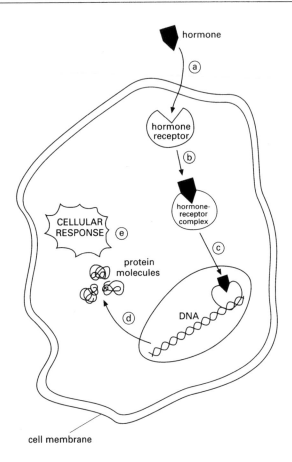

Fig. 4.4. How the direct gene mechanism of hormone action works. (a) A fat-soluble hormone enters the cell. (b) It binds to a receptor to form a hormone–receptor complex. (c) This passes through to the nucleus and activates specific genes. (d) Protein synthesis occurs. (e) The proteins produce a cellular response.

hormone is the production of new protein molecules of a particular type within the cell.

A quick tour of the endocrine system

The pituitary gland is often called the master gland of the endocrine system; in fact this title rightly belongs to the hypothalamus, which is the true control centre of the body. The front of the pituitary is connected to the hypothalamus by a blood vessel, while the back makes a connection through the nervous system. Both allow signals from the hypothalamus to dictate the release of a number of pituitary hormones, all of them peptides.

For instance, antidiuretic hormone (ADH) aids water balance in the body. It acts on the kidney, where it decreases urine output. Increased ADH secretion is part of the body's emergency response to a fall in circulating blood volume, which can occur in severe haemorrhage, burns, or with vomiting and diarrhoea. If the situation goes uncorrected, the organs will be deprived of oxygen and will fail rapidly. Decreasing urine output is one way of keeping the blood volume up.

Another important pituitary hormone is growth hormone which acts on all parts of the body. It does exactly what the name suggests, and is active mainly in childhood and adolescence. Its main effects are on the long bones, and on muscle mass. Oxytocin and prolactin are active in pregnancy and childbirth. The former causes contractions of the uterus and milk expulsion, while the latter is responsible for milk production.

The remaining pituitary hormones act on other endocrine glands. Thyroid stimulating hormone has already been mentioned; corticotropin acts on the adrenals to get them to produce glucocorticoid hormones in response to stress. Finally, the pituitary plays a key role in regulation of the menstrual cycle by the production of follicle stimulating hormone (FSH) and luteinising hormone (LH) under the direction of gonaderelin which is released from the hypothalamus (the menstrual cycle will be discussed in more detail later).

Thyroid hormones, as mentioned above, speed up the production of energy and oxygen consumption in cells. They also speed up the heart rate and have several other functions. They are the only body chemicals that contain the element iodine and thyroid hormone deficiency may occur in inland areas where the iodine content of the water is low. It is rare in coastal areas, where iodine levels in the water tend to be high. The thyroid also produces calcitonin and parathormone which control the levels of calcium and phosphate in the blood, moving it to and from bone as necessary.

Moving down the body, the adrenal glands produce two groups of steroid hormones – the glucocorticoids, and the mineralocorticoids. The glucocorticoids are cortisol, corticosterone and cortisone. They mobilise energy resources in times of physical or emotional stress by promoting certain biochemical reactions; they break down proteins and fats into amino acids and fatty acids respectively. Both can be used to build emergency supplies of glucose in a process called gluconeogenesis to help meet the demands of a stressful situation. The glucocorticoids also have a powerful anti-inflammatory effect, which is the basis for their therapeutic use (to be discussed later).

The adrenals produce two other stress hormones, noradrenaline and adrenaline. Unlike the glucocorticoids, these are produced directly in response to stress – without the intervention of the hypothalamus or pituitary. Both put the body into a 'flight or fight' mode by triggering a number of physiological events. Adrenaline acts on the cardiovascular system, increasing the heart rate, opening up the blood vessels and increasing blood pressure. At the same time respiratory rate goes up. All of this ensures that the muscles get extra oxygen. The cells are primed to consume oxygen more rapidly, generating extra biochemical energy for the response to stress. The muscles get less fatigued, and the blood clots more easily in case of injury. The effects of noradrenaline are broadly similar. Unlike the corticosteroids, these are catecholamines and act on receptors outside their target cells. There are two types of receptor for adrenaline and noradrenaline on their target organs, such as the heart. Each can bind both hormones, but alpha-receptors tend to respond mainly to noradrenaline, and beta-receptors to adrenaline.

A full-blown stress response is obviously life-saving under conditions of extreme danger – such as being chased by a tiger. But for most people these days, this level of response is rarely necessary. While an adrenaline 'rush' may create a pleasurable 'high', in the long term stress hormones can damage the body and mind, leading to heart disease, high blood pressure and chronic anxiety symptoms. Recent research, by scientists at Washington University School of Medicine, also suggests that chronically high levels of cortisol may shrink the hippocampus, the part of the brain concerned with memory and learning.

The pancreatic peptide hormones insulin and glucagon act in tandem to control the amount of glucose in the blood (sometimes known as blood sugar). The human engine runs on glucose, which is its main fuel. To keep running smoothly, the blood sugar – the level of glucose in the blood – must stay within the range of 70 to 100 milligrams per 100 millilitres. This gives the organs of the body a steady fuel supply to provide the energy for their various activities. Typically humans refuel three or four times a day, taking in carbohydrate foods like bread, pasta and potatoes which the digestive system breaks down into glucose.

Careful budgeting is needed so that the excess glucose in the blood after a meal is stored away, ready for release when blood sugar falls – either overnight or after exercise. Suppose you have just eaten a lunch of soup, bread, pasta, and fruit. Within the hour, glucose floods the blood stream. The organs take what they need, but the rest must be stored for later. High blood sugar is the chemical signal which releases insulin from the pancreas. The insulin heads for cells in the liver and the muscles, where it locks onto insulin receptors on the cell membranes. This interaction triggers various chemical reactions inside the cells, mediated by cAMP (see Fig. 4.3 again). These reactions involve the uptake of glucose from the blood into the cells, followed by its conversion into a stored form called glycogen. The blood sugar then falls to a normal value.

Now suppose you play a vigorous game of tennis a couple of hours after that lunch. The muscle cells are burning up glucose at more than their normal rate to keep the action going. Eventually blood sugar begins to fall. Now glucagon – insulin's opposite number – is released from the pancreas. It targets the muscle cells, acting – like insulin – on a receptor protein. This triggers the breakdown of glycogen within the cells, providing them with much-needed glucose and raising blood sugar to a normal level. Glucagon can also create glucose from other sources such as amino acids, and lactic acid, again by acting upon receptors on cell membranes. In short, when the blood sugar is too low, the action of glucagon restores it to a normal value.

The testes makes the male sex hormone testosterone which acts under the influence of FSH and LH to stimulate production of sperm. It is also responsible for development of the male sexual organs, the production of facial and pubic hair, the deepening of the voice, and sexual behaviour. The corresponding female hormones are oestrogen and progesterone which are produced by the ovary – again under the influence of FSH and LH – and are responsible for the development of the breasts and the control of the menstrual cycle. All the sex hormones are steroids.

Finally, the pineal gland produces melatonin at night. Its production is inhibited by light and it may play some role in sleep–wake cycles. Recently there has been much interest in the potential of melatonin to delay the onset of the ageing process. (The therapeutic uses of melatonin are discussed further in Chapter 10.)

Hormone drugs

Millions of people take hormone drugs. Some are natural hormones, like the body's own chemical messengers, while others are synthetic derivatives.

They may be prescribed to remedy a hormone deficiency, to interfere with naturally occurring hormonal responses, or to treat diseases which have nothing to do with hormones.

One important characteristic of some hormone drugs is that they may be taken for many years, like the contraceptive pill, or for life, as with insulin. They may also be taken by healthy people; oral contraceptives and hormone replacement therapy fall into this category, as do fertility drugs. Therefore there is always intense interest in any reports of any new side effects, or long-term effects, of hormonal medicines.

Hormones for deficiency diseases

Diabetes mellitus (usually just called diabetes) is the most common hormonal deficiency disease. Thirty million people worldwide (750,000 in the UK) suffer from diabetes, a condition resulting from insulin deficiency or resistance. There are two forms of diabetes. In type I diabetes, the pancreas fails to produce any insulin. This condition occurs more often in young people. Type II diabetes is three times commoner than type I and occurs when insulin is produced normally, but cannot be used by the body. This so-called insulin resistance is often associated with obesity. Type II diabetes appears to be on the increase; a recent study suggested it doubled in incidence in the 15 years to 1989.

If an untreated diabetic eats a high-carbohydrate lunch, excess glucose stays in the blood because there is no insulin to push it into the liver for storage. Glucose is a diuretic; it increases the output of urine. In fact the term diabetes comes from the Greek word for siphon, referring to one of the main symptoms, which is excessive urination. After a meal the excess blood sugar is excreted in the diabetic's urine instead of being stored for later use by cells. (The word mellitus, which means honey in Latin, was added to the name in the 17th century when physicians discovered that diabetic urine tastes sweet – this low-tech test was diagnostic of the condition.) Eventually the cells become starved of glucose and, in a desperate attempt to obtain fuel, they start to break down fat instead. This process gives rise to poisonous by-products called ketones, which can bring on a life-threatening diabetic coma.

Diabetes was first described in Egypt in around 1500 BC. Doctors tried to treat it with a mixture of bones, ground earth, wheat and lead – but to no avail. The condition was usually fatal and remained mysterious until the late 19th century, when it was shown that removal of the pancreas caused diabetes. Insulin itself was discovered by the Canadian surgeon Frederick Banting and his partner Charles Best. They tried it out on a diabetic dog called Marjorie and restored her to health. The first person to receive insulin, in 1922, was a 14-year-old boy dying of diabetes called Leonard Thompson. The drug saved his life.

Today type I diabetics can control their condition with daily injections of insulin. The aim of the treatment is to mimic normal insulin secretion which consists of a small baseline level to deal with small fluctuations in blood sugar, and a surge after a meal to tidy away the excess glucose that floods the bloodstream. There are short, medium and long-term acting insulins (depending on the particle size of the drug) and most people manage their diabetes with an injection of a mixture of short and longer-acting insulins twice a day, given before breakfast and before their evening meal.

Diabetes is associated with long-term complications such as blindness, kidney disease, heart disease, and stroke. Research has shown that these are reduced if the diabetic adopts a more intensive treatment programme of three or more injections a day, coupled with four glucose monitoring assessments by measuring blood sugar or testing for the presence of sugar in the urine.

Traditionally insulin has been extracted from animal pancreas, and many diabetics have spent years taking pork or beef insulin. Nowadays most insulin is made by genetic engineering and is derived from the human insulin gene (more about genetically engineered drugs in Chapter 11). Human insulin differs from beef and pork insulins by two and one amino acids respectively. It is more easily absorbed by the body. Some diabetics have complained that the switch to human insulin has made them less aware of the warning signs of a hypoglycaemic episode (a 'hypo'). This happens when the insulin makes the blood sugar go to too low a level, perhaps because the person has missed a meal. Symptoms include faintness, irritability, seizures and even coma. However, clinical studies have not borne out these observations.

Another hormone which is now produced by genetic engineering is human growth hormone. Lack of growth hormone can lead to short stature, and treatment with it can encourage normal growth. The hormone used to be extracted from human pituitary glands and in a few cases, Creutzfeld-Jakob disease was transmitted in this way. With the genetically engineered hormone, there is no such risk.

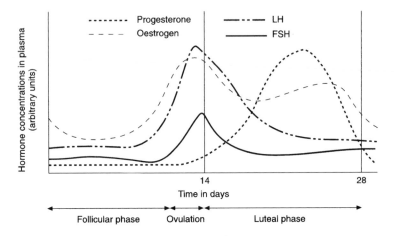

Fig. 4.5. Hormonal variations during the menstrual cycle. Gonadotrophin releasing hormone (GnRH), from the hypothalamus, stimulates the production of follicle stimulating hormone (FSH) and luteinising hormone (LH) from the pituitary. FSH promotes ripening of follicles – one of which releases an egg during ovulation. LH turns this empty follicle into the corpus luteum which secretes progesterone during the second half of the cycle. Oestrogen, produced from ripening follicles, both inhibits further production of FSH during the follicular phase and triggers a surge of LH just before ovulation. Falling levels of oestrogen and progesterone towards the end of the cycle cause production of FSH and LH to rise again, ready to repeat the cycle. Hormonal drugs interfere with this cycle in a number of ways. Oral contraceptives maintain high oestrogen and progesterone levels so FSH and LH are not secreted, mimicking the luteal phase and inhibiting ovulation. Fertility drugs stimulate FSH or LH. The abortion pill suppresses progesterone, while HRT mimics the oestrogen and progesterone levels of a menstruating woman, but without FSH or LH.

Sex hormones

Intervention in the menstrual cycle has allowed the development of three types of drug which have given women the potential to control their biology – oral contraceptives, fertility drugs and hormone replacement therapy (HRT).

The menstrual cycle is the result of a hormonal interplay between the brain, the ovaries, and the womb (Fig. 4.5). The events taking place in the ovary can be divided into three phases. If the first day of menstrual bleeding is taken as day 1, then the follicular phase typically runs from day 1 to day

10. The hypothalamus releases pulses of gonadotrophin releasing hormone (GnRH) which directs production of FSH and LH from the pituitary. Under the influence of these hormones several of the follicles – fluid-filled sacs which contain an immature egg – on each ovary begin to mature. Eventually one of these follicles dominates and forms a mature egg, ready for possible fertilisation.

At the same time, the follicles start to secrete oestrogen. This inhibits the production of FSH, stopping any of the other follicles from maturing. The follicles become more sensitive to FSH and LH and output of oestrogen rises. Higher oestrogen levels eventually trigger a surge of LH which begins on about day 10. Now the cycle enters the ovulation phase which involves release of the mature egg, which travels towards the Fallopian tube.

The empty follicle develops into a structure called the corpus luteum, under the influence of LH, and the last 14 days of the cycle – a phase which is invariable in length in contrast to the first two phases – are known as the luteal phase. The corpus luteum produces oestrogen and progesterone, both of which inhibit the production of further FSH and LH; these are no longer required, since ovulation has already occurred. But from day 22, the corpus luteum starts to regress, and oestrogen and progesterone levels drop. FSH and LH levels begin to rise once more, and from day 28 the cycle will repeat itself – if pregnancy has not occurred.

Meanwhile in the uterus, menstrual bleeding stops around day 5 and oestrogen starts to prepare the lining of the womb for a possible pregnancy, increasing its thickness so that nutrients can be carried through the blood to the developing embryo. When progesterone secretion occurs, it continues preparing the womb for pregnancy. If fertilisation does not occur, levels of oestrogen and progesterone drop and the womb lining breaks down and is shed during the next menstrual period.

Oral contraceptives Oral contraceptives contain synthetic oestrogen and progesterone and they are among the most widely prescribed drugs in the world. They first became available in the 1960s and are now taken by 63 million women worldwide. Taken correctly, the Pill is at least 99 per cent effective – that is, of 100 women taking the Pill one, at most, will get pregnant every year.

The hormones in oral contraceptives mimic the hormonal situation of early pregnancy, where levels of oestrogen and progesterone are high enough to inhibit production of FSH and LH and so stop ovulation. The Pill has other contraceptive effects; it thickens cervical mucus, making it harder for sperm to travel to the Fallopian tubes and meet the egg, and it makes the endometrium (the lining of the womb) unreceptive to the implantation of a fertilised egg.

There are many different formulations of the Pill. Combined oral contraceptives contain both an oestrogen-like component and a progestogen (the name given to progesterone and synthetic derivatives that act in a similar way). Ethinyloestradiol is the commonest oestrogen used in oral contraceptives, while levonorgestrel is the commonest progestogen. The earlier 'first generation' Pills, available in the 1970s, had a much higher hormone content than the 'second generation' Pills, which were formulated from the discovery that a lower hormone dose had a similar contraceptive effect but with fewer side effects. More recently so-called 'third generation' Pills have been developed which contain the progesterones desogestrel, gestodene and nor-gestimate. These are thought to be less likely to lead to serious (but still rare) adverse effects such as heart attack or stroke than the older Pills. Some women experience fewer side effects on the newer Pills.

There are also progesterone-only Pills, which are often prescribed to older women, or women who cannot tolerate taking oestrogen. These do not completely inhibit ovulation and rely on the thickening of cervical mucus for their contraceptive effect. There are also three-month depot injections of levonorgestrel, and an implant, Norplant, which lasts for five years. Recently on the market is Mirena, a cervical implant of levonorgestrel which acts like a cross between an intrauterine device and an oral contraceptive (and is known as an intrauterine system or IUS); because the hormone acts locally and does not get into the system there should be fewer side effects and long-term effects. Mirena gives three years of continuous contraceptive protection and is about as effective as female sterilisation. It is also fully reversible.

It is also possible to use oral contraceptives to prevent conception after unprotected intercourse, using the 'morning after' Pill. This consists of a relatively high dose of ethinyloestradiol and levonorgestrel given in two stages, twelve hours apart. The first dose has to be taken within 72 hours of intercourse. Depending on where the woman is in her cycle, it either stops ovulation or prevents implantation; the method is up to 96 per cent effective in preventing pregnancy.

Sex hormones are powerful chemicals; women taking them have to balance their individual benefit/risk equations. There are a number of side effects which will soon become apparent: irregular bleeding, weight gain, headache, nausea, yeast infections and depression affect 20 to 30 per cent of women on the Pill. Sometimes these side effects fade with time, or can be dealt with by using a different formulation of Pill. But 10 to 15 per cent stop taking the Pill because of side effects. The Pill also interacts with several other drugs including some antibiotics and anti-epilepsy drugs. These inter-actions may make the Pill less effective.

As for the long-term effects of the Pill, it is difficult to come to firm conclusions because the formulations of the drugs have changed so much over the last 20 years. So while a woman could be taking hormones for 20 years or more, it is most unlikely she will remain on the first Pill she was prescribed, which 'moves the goal posts' of any clinical studies. Research that has been done centres around two main concerns – cardiovascular disease, and cancer. These risks come about because some progesterones can have an adverse effect on the lipid profile in the blood, which predisposes to cardiovascular problems, while oestrogen can cause breast tissue to divide abnormally, possibly leading to a tumour. Oestrogen also makes the blood more likely to clot.

High levels of oestrogen during pregnancy lead to an increased risk of deep vein thrombosis (DVT) in which a blood clot forms in a vein in the leg. DVT is not dangerous in itself, but there is a one to two per cent chance of the clot breaking off and moving to the lungs, heart or brain and forming a potentially fatal obstruction called an embolism. The risk of DVT in pregnancy is 60 per 100,000 women, and in women who are neither pregnant nor on the Pill it is 5 per 100,000. Going on the Pill increases this risk three times to 15 per 100,000, while recent research suggested that third generation Pills containing desogestrel and gestodene doubled the risk of DVT again to an incidence of 30 per 100,000. In response to this news, many women stopped taking the Pill, without first seeking medical advice, and became pregnant thereby doubling their risk of DVT (from 30 to 60 in 100,000).

Undoubtedly a few of these women would have developed DVT had they carried on taking the Pill. Most would have been perfectly all right. The good news is that it is now possible to identify well over half of those at risk of DVT by genetic screening. Over the last few years, researchers in the Netherlands and Sweden have shown that up to 33 per cent of people with DVT carry a mutation in a blood clotting protein called Factor V. This mutation makes the blood more likely to clot, and it is common among the North European population, occurring with a frequency ranging from 3–25 per cent. Although it would probably not be cost-effective to screen every woman wanting to take the Pill for this mutation, there is a case for it if she has a first-degree relative under 45 with DVT. And if she does carry the mutation, she should not take any kind of Pill.

There are other women who should never take the Pill. A responsible doctor will not prescribe it to anyone with existing heart disease, for example, or to a heavy smoker. For other women it is a matter of weighing up the risks and benefits. There are good reasons for women not to abandon the third generation Pills. As mentioned above, they are less likely to lead to other cardiovascular problems such as heart disease and stroke. These are more likely to be fatal than DVT. A woman who, on balance, is more likely to be at risk of cardiovascular problems than DVT should really opt for a third generation Pill. But some risk factors, like obesity, predispose to both cardiovascular disease *and* DVT. In such cases, a woman will need very careful counselling before coming to a decision.

As far as cancer is concerned, there is good evidence that the Pill actually decreases the risk of ovarian and endometrial cancer . There may be an increase in cervical cancer, especially in women who started the Pill at a young age. This, however, may not be due to the Pill itself but may have more to do with the lack of barrier protection against sexually transmitted viruses, such as papillomavirus, which are now known to be linked to cervical cancer. And frequent changes of sexual partner makes transmission of cancer-causing viruses more likely.

On breast cancer the latest research, which looked at 150,000 Pill users, concluded that whilst taking the Pill women run a 25 per cent increased risk of breast cancer. In the ten years after stopping the Pill, the risk is an extra 16 per cent in the first five years, and this drops to one per cent in the next five years. Beyond 10 years the risk is no greater than if the women had never taken the Pill. Further, the cancers diagnosed in Pill users and ex-Pill users tended to be localised in the breast. And those diagnosed more than ten years after stopping the Pill tend also to be less advanced than those in women who have never used the Pill.

Also in the pipeline are hormonal contraceptives for men. The 'male Pill' is a progestogen which tells the pituitary to stop producing sperm. The main side effect is a decline in testosterone, which is reversed by periodic injections of the hormones. Clinical trials have shown it to be as effective as the female Pill, and it should be on the market before the end of the century.

However, there is room for further development. Carl Djerassi of Stanford University, the chemist who pioneered the Pill, has recently criticised drug companies for not getting more involved in contraceptive research. According to Djerassi, a contraceptive vaccine or a once-a-month menstruation-inducing or anti-implantation Pill would be far better than current options. He accuses the industry of cold-shouldering these new ideas because they would result in far cheaper drugs (one pill a month is almost certain to be more cost-effective than one a day) and so slice into profits from this enormous worldwide market.

Fertility treatment Around one couple in six is infertile – that is, they do not conceive within a year of trying for a baby. The commonest causes include low sperm count, failure to ovulate, and blocked Fallopian tubes. Drugs which intervene in the menstrual cycle are commonly used to treat the latter two conditions.

Lack of ovulation accounts for around 20 per cent of all infertility. It can be treated by clomiphene, an oestrogen antagonist. This stops the feedback effect of oestrogen on the hypothalamus, and enables it to release FSH and LH, which will trigger ovulation. Another option is to give GnRH to stimulate production of FSH and LH; usually the woman is given a syringe pump to administer pulses of GnRH like those naturally produced by the body. FSH and LH can also be used directly; they are synthesised by genetic engineering, or are extracted from the urine of post-menopausal women (human menopausal gonadotrophin), or pregnant women (human chorionic gonadotrophin). Any one of these drug treatments should stimulate ovulation.

Sometimes a woman ovulates normally, but conception cannot occur because the tubes are blocked, so the egg cannot meet the sperm in the usual place. In such cases, which account for another 20 per cent of infertility, *in vitro* fertilisation (IVF) might be the answer. In IVF, sperm and egg are extracted from the man and woman, and mixed in a glass dish to fertilise. The embryos are then replaced in the womb.

There are two ways of doing IVF. In natural cycle IVF no drugs are used, but the woman's LH levels are monitored by 12-hourly plasma assays (this involves a blood test). Once the surge that precedes ovulation occurs, the ripening follicle is punctured to 'capture' the egg, which is then fertilised and replaced in the womb. The 'take home baby' rate (live births per treatment cycle) is typically only six per cent with natural cycle IVF, because the egg often escapes from the ovary before retrieval, and only one embryo is replaced. Although natural IVF is easier on the woman physically, because it is drug-free, it is not much used because of the low success rate.

More common is superovulation IVF where a combination of drugs is used to control the cycle so that egg retrieval is more precise. The drugs also allow the production of several eggs in one cycle. First GnRH is 'down-regulated' by a GnRH agonist such as nafarelin or buserelin, which are administered as a nasal spray. Once the pituitary action is turned off, the woman is, temporarily, in a state of artificial menopause. Then her cycle is restored by synthetic gonadotrophins such as Pergonal or Humegon which stand in for FSH and LH. Egg retrieval is guided by ultrasound, and several – up to ten, typically – are fertilised. The chances of success are maximised because the embryologist selects the best-looking embryos under a microscope. Up to three embryos are then replaced in the womb. At this stage injections or suppositories of progesterone are given until pregnancy is confirmed (or not) to induce the uterine lining to proliferate ready for implantation (as it normally would do after ovulation). The success rate with superovulation is up to 25 per cent.

The abortion pill Mifepristone is a progesterone antagonist which has been developed as RU486, the so-called 'abortion pill'. Since progesterone is essential for implantation RU486 works by blocking its action. The drug is usually given by mouth within 63 days of a missed period and is followed by a synthetic prostaglandin 36 to 48 hours later. The prostaglandin is a hormone which has a number of effects, including cervical dilation and uterine contraction – so in this context it works with the mifepristone by expelling the contents of the womb. The abortion normally occurs within hours of administration of the prostaglandin and only a tiny minority of women will need surgery to complete removal of the foetus.

Gemeprost is currently the prostaglandin of choice, but it has the drawback of being expensive and difficult to transport and store. Of the 30 million abortions carried out each year worldwide, a substantial number are in developing countries. A recent report on the effectiveness of an alternative prostaglandin, misoprostol, which is cheaper and easier to handle, opens up the possibility of the medical abortion becoming more widely available. However, the abortion pill just has not taken off. In the UK its availability in the health service is patchy, while it accounts for only two per cent of terminations in the private sector. Now RU 486 is to be withdrawn by its manufacturers, almost certainly because of political pressure from anti-abortion campaigners who have grabbed the high moral ground on this important women's health issue.

Hormone replacement therapy A woman's fertility begins to wane, typically, when she is in her 30s, and the menopause – the last menstrual period –

will occur some time between age 45 and 55 (average age around 52). Fluctuating, and falling, oestrogen levels around the menopause may give rise to a number of physical and psychological symptoms. Seventy per cent of all menopausal women suffer vasomotor symptoms which are due to the effects of oestrogen on the dilation and constriction of the blood vessels; these include hot flushes, sweating, insomnia and dizziness. In a quarter of women these symptoms may last for over five years. Other common symptoms include vaginal dryness, cystitis, and depression.

Treatment of menopausal symptoms with hormones began with Brooklyn gynaecologist Robert Wilson's book *Forever Feminine*, in which he advocated the use of Premarin, an oestrogen preparation from the urine of pregnant mares. The idea is quite simple – supply the hormones that are being lost and restore the pre-menopausal state (but without the risk of pregnancy, because the pituitary hormones are not replaced).

Over the years it has become apparent that replacing lost oestrogen may help with women's long-term health problems too. Natural oestrogen appears to offer some protection against coronary heart disease (CHD). At age 60, the rates of CHD in women and men are the same, while before the menopause they are much lower – by around 50 per cent – in women. Taking oestrogen lowers the risk of CHD by 50 per cent and of stroke by 20 per cent. The effect seems to come from the effect of oestrogen on the lipid profile; more of this in the next chapter, but in brief, oestrogen increases high density lipoprotein ('good' cholesterol) and thereby decreases the incidence of fatty deposits in the coronary arteries, which can lead to impaired blood flow to the heart.

Oestrogen also appears to prevent bone loss if it is taken long-term (more than five years); ten years after menopause most women have lost 15 per cent of their bone mass. The condition is known as osteoporosis and leads to brittle bones which are more likely to fracture. However, osteoporosis can also be prevented by adequate intake of calcium, weight-bearing exercise such as walking, and other drugs such as bisphosphonates. There may be more to osteoporosis than oestrogen. While it is commoner in women, it is on the increase in both men and women – who are three times more likely to fracture their hips than people of comparable age were 30 years ago.

Recent research also suggests that HRT can cut the risk of developing Alzheimer's disease (AD), a brain disorder characterised by memory loss and personality change (of which more in Chapter 8). In a group of over 1000 American women, 6 per cent of those who had taken oestrogen developed AD during the study compared to 16 per cent of those who had never taken HRT. And women who had taken HRT appeared to develop AD at a later age. The longer they had taken oestrogen the more likely they were to be protected from AD. No one is quite sure of the nature of the protective effects – but oestrogen increases cerebral blood flow and protects the brain from the harmful effects of glucocorticoid hormones. Many women on HRT claim it does improve their memory – which fits the clinical studies. More recent research suggests that oestrogen has a profoundly beneficial effect on brain cells in both women and men – it acts as an antioxidant, strengthens neuronal memory circuits, and increases the levels of the neurotransmitter acectylcholine, which is deficient in AD.

In the 1970s it was found that women who took oestrogen alone in HRT ran a greater than normal risk of contracting endometrial cancer. Nowadays it is given with a progestogen (so-called 'opposed' oestrogen). It is available as a tablet, skin patch, implant or cream – depending upon the duration and reason for its use. Women who have had a hysterectomy can taken unopposed oestrogen. The oestrogen used is oestradiol, a natural form of oestrogen which does not carry a thrombosis risk. The progestogen is dydrogesterone, which does give a monthly 'bleed' like a period. However, there are now preparations which avoid this.

HRT is associated with a number of side effects such as headaches, mood changes and dizziness. The progestogen component may lead to bloating, cramps, breast tenderness and nausea. It may make depression worse in women who have previously suffered from premenstrual syndrome. The take-up of HRT in Britain among the general population is relatively low at 15 per cent and less than five per cent of these women take it for more than two years. However, a survey of female GPs in the UK paints a different picture; the majority of these women opt for HRT. This ties in with a recent report from Sweden. While only 24 per cent of menopausal Swedish women take HRT, 86 per cent of female gynaecologists take it, and a similar percentage of male gynaecologists' wives. The corresponding figures for Swedish GPs are around 10 per cent lower. This strongly suggests that, influenced mainly by clinical evidence, medics opt for HRT for themselves while their patients may be put off by media scare stories. Only time will tell who made the right decision.

Taking HRT long-term poses a subtle cost–benefits problem, which is similar to the oral contraceptive dilemma. Oestrogen alone leads to a 30 per cent increase in breast cancer, rising to 50 per cent if it is taken for more than 10 years. It was hoped that this risk would decrease with the addition of a progestogen to HRT. These hopes have not really been borne out by research. Oestrogen decreases the risk of heart disease and stroke, and these are five times more common than breast and endometrial cancer, whose risk is increased by oestrogen. On a population-wide basis, the answer may be clear – menopausal women should take HRT. For the individual woman, the decision is more complex and depends upon how long she takes HRT, when she begins it, and – most importantly – her family history and individual risk factors.

What remains uncertain is how long the protective effects in cardiovascular disease persist after stopping HRT, and how long the corresponding risk of breast cancer remains. Since the average woman spends around a third of her life in the post-menopausal stage, whether or not to take HRT is a decision as important as that on which type of contraception she should use.

This decision should be easier in the future. First, there are big prospective studies underway which should provide some answers on the risks of HRT. A European trial involving 30,000 women has just been launched. Half will take HRT and the other half a placebo. They will be monitored for several years for heart disease, osteoporosis, breast cancer and psychological health. The first results, on the effect of HRT on heart disease and stroke, are expected by 2012. The European study complements the ongoing Women's Health Initiative study of menopausal women in the US.

Second, drug development should produce oestrogen-type drugs which offer all the benefits without the risks. Oestrogens are notoriously 'two-faced' – as you might expect from such powerful hormones. Tamoxifen, for example, which is given to women with, or at risk of, breast cancer, will block the effect of oestrogen in breast tissue. But it acts like oestrogen in the womb, putting women on tamoxifen at risk of uterine cancer. So anyone considering tamoxifen has a tricky cost–benefit equation to weigh up.

However, there is increasing interest in oestrogens that are more specific in their actions. It has long been known that oriental women have a far lower incidence of breast cancer than women in the West, and one reason could be their intake of natural oestrogens from soy products in their diet. These plant oestrogens, the isoflavones, have not been much studied as yet, but could provide a source of safer forms of HRT.

Already a recent report from scientists at the Lilly Research Laboratories in Indianapolis highlights a new synthetic oestrogen called raloxifene, which appears to have very desirable properties. Like tamoxifen, it blocks oestrogen in breast tissue but acts like oestrogen in the bone, increasing bone density. But it does not stimulate growth of uterine tissue because raloxifene does not interact with the same genes as do oestrogen and tamoxifen. So it does not take the brakes off genes that might lead to cancer. This opens up the idea of designing oestrogens that are very specific as to their effects within the body. If this work is successful, it should offer women a wider range of options for HRT and decrease the risk of adverse effects.

Hormones for non-hormonal diseases

Corticosteroids such as prednisolone are widely used to treat inflammatory diseases such as arthritis, ulcerative colitis, asthma and allergic diseases such as eczema. However, steroids are powerful drugs; sometimes they are given as local injections (such as into an arthritic knee) or as creams to avoid their getting into the circulation. They cause a characteristic 'moon' face swelling by moving body fat to the facial region. They may also lead to high blood pressure, and because they damp down the inflammatory response, which is part of the immune system, they also increase susceptibility to infection.

Steroid hormones have both immediate and long-term effects on body chemistry. Even in a medical context, problems can occur. Some people take steroids for non-medical reasons. Because the male sex hormones can build muscle and stamina, they have been popular among athletes as a way of improving sporting performance for some years.

Anabolic steroids are drugs which resemble testosterone. When a boy reaches adolescence testosterone is produced by the testicles and has a number of effects on his body. The androgenic or masculinising effects of testosterone include the development of the sexual organs – the penis, scrotum and prostate gland – as well as the appearance of body hair and the deepening of the voice. Testosterone also has anabolic or tissue-building effects; it makes boys taller and broader, increasing the mass of their muscles. Until adolescence girls are often taller than boys. Then, thanks to testosterone, boys shoot past them. Athletes are interested in the anabolic effects of testosterone; if they take anabolic steroids the drugs enhance performance by building muscle mass, strength and endurance.

Two Austrian physiologists, Oskar Zoth and Fritz Pregl, were the first to promote the idea of using anabolic steroids in sport. In 1896 they injected themselves with extract of bull's testicles and measured the strength of their middle fingers. But it was not until 1935 that testosterone was shown to be the active ingredient in this extract. By the 1940s the use of testosterone – and, later, related drugs – was widespread among bodybuilders. The practice spread to people involved in field and track events, football, and many other sports.

Sports authorities at all levels have banned the use of anabolic steroids and other drugs, arguing that they give competitors an unfair advantage. The 1976 Montreal Olympics saw the first official tests for anabolic steroids. The drugs break down in the body to give substances which can be detected in the urine. The urine tests have become more reliable and sensitive over the years, and many high-profile athletes have been caught out by them.

According to scientific evidence, the main effect on the body of the anabolic steroids used in sport is to build muscle mass. This is only really useful in sports such as weight lifting and American football, where muscle bulk is crucial for success. But anabolic steroids have psychological effects too. They increase aggression and self-confidence and give a feeling of well-being. Experiments show this helps athletes train harder, and recover more quickly from a punishing schedule. Anabolic steroids are also being used increasingly by young men who want a more muscular, tough, and masculine body image. Steroids are powerful drugs. Even without urine tests, it is often possible to tell who is taking anabolic steroids because they cause side effects such as acne, infertility, weight gain and mood swings. Women athletes who take them may become more masculine, and develop deep voices and excess body hair.

Hormones have caused a cultural revolution by allowing women to take control of their fertility. And the beneficial effects of female sex hormones – as HRT – on cardiovascular disease highlights one of the main concerns of the 20th century. The drugs used to treat cardiovascular disease, and to protect against it, will be looked at in the next chapter.

5

Cardiovascular drugs: protecting the heart and brain

Cardiovascular (CV) disease, the name given to all those conditions which affect the heart and circulation, has become an increasingly important target for the pharmaceutical industry over the last 20 years or so. Nine of the top 20 best-selling drugs are for treating CV disease (Table 1). This is hardly surprising, since the market is enormous.

The two main areas of CV disease are coronary heart disease (CHD) and stroke. In the UK, CV disease accounts for around 300,000 deaths every year – nearly half of the total number of deaths. Half of these deaths are from CHD, and a quarter are from stroke (the rest are due to related conditions).

However, the mortality from CHD has been falling in the UK since the late 1970s. Today slightly more people die of some form of cancer than of CHD. A similar downward trend is seen in many other countries in the world (Fig. 5.1), especially in the United States. Britain still has one of the highest rates of CHD in the world, exceeded only by figures for Eastern Europe and the former Soviet Union, where – alarmingly – rates are actually increasing. Coronary heart disease levels are particularly low in some Mediterranean countries such as France and Italy, and lowest of all in Japan. No one is sure of the reasons for these various trends, and the differences in CHD rates between different countries, but they reflect the impact of an interplay of both lifestyle factors and genetics. Cardiovascular drugs work alongside lifestyle changes to improve the outlook for those affected by CV disease, while genetic research may, in the future, pinpoint those who stand to benefit most from their use (see also Chapter 11).

Atherosclerosis sets the scene for cardiovascular disease

The seeds of CV disease are often sown many years before any symptoms appear, when fatty deposits called plaque start to build up on the inner walls

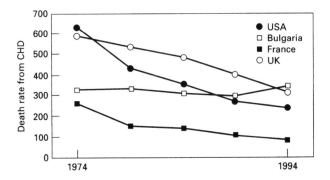

Fig. 5.1. Death rates from coronary heart disease in different countries. Death rates for men aged between 35–74 per 100,000 population from 1972–1992 (vertical axis) shown over the 20-year period from 1974–94 (horizontal points shown at 5-year periods). Some countries show a downward trend (UK, USA). In some (Bulgaria, and other Eastern European countries not shown) the trend is upwards. Some countries, such as France (and Mexico, Greece and Italy – not shown), have relatively low rates of coronary heart disease. Data: British Heart Foundation.

of the arteries. With time, a plaque narrows, or even blocks, the arteries, leading to a condition called atherosclerosis. The condition is worsened by the natural hardening of the arteries, known as arteriosclerosis, which occurs with age. Blood flows more slowly through narrowed arteries, and is more likely to form a clot known as a thrombosis, particularly if a plaque cracks or ruptures. Should the thrombosis occur in an artery serving the heart or brain, it will probably result in a potentially fatal heart attack or stroke.

Hardened and narrowed arteries can occur anywhere in the body, but the coronary arteries, the aorta and the carotid arteries in the head are most often affected. Atherosclerosis can only be reversed at a very early stage, where so-called 'fatty streaks' – the precursor of plaque – have developed on the inner lining of the arteries. These fatty streaks have been observed in school-age children, showing that damage does indeed start early in life. The fatty streaks may disappear, but once plaques have developed, self-help and medical treatment can only stop them getting worse. There are no drugs which can stop the formation of atherosclerotic plaque, but lipid-lowering drugs (discussed in a later section) may stop it developing.

No one knows what causes the deposition of plaque. One leading theory is that it starts off with an injury to the endothelial cells which line the artery walls. This initial injury could be caused by high cholesterol concentrations, infection (see also Chapter 3), or cigarette smoke. In a classic inflammation response, white blood cells called macrophages then migrate to the site of the injury and begin to ingest cholesterol molecules (which they mark out as being 'foreign'). Cholesterol-filled macrophages form structures called foam cells, which tend to adhere to the artery walls, creating a fatty streak. Now the body may try to heal the wound by laying down scar tissue, made of muscle cells, on top of the fatty streak. Maybe the process will stop here – but if someone continues to smoke, or eat a fatty diet, the inflammatory process will become chronic and the lesion will expand into a true athero-sclerotic plaque.

When disaster strikes – heart attacks and stroke

Blood clotting has obvious survival value to animals with a circulatory system. Injury to a blood vessel triggers a cascade of biochemical reactions which culminates in the transformation of a protein called fibrinogen into a thread-like protein called fibrin. At the same time, red blood cells called platelets clump together and get tangled up in the fibrin threads, forming a clot over the site of the wound. Clots which stop blood escaping are essential; clots which form in a vessel and stop the blood moving are life-threatening.

The usual cause of a heart attack is blockage of one of the coronary arteries by a blood clot. The blockage is known as a coronary thrombosis and it cuts off the supply of blood to the heart. The resulting lack of oxygen damages, and may even kill, an area of the heart tissue. The damaged area is known as an infarct (the clinical term for heart attack is myocardial infarction; the myocardium is the name for the heart muscle). The amount of damage caused by a heart attack depends upon how big the infarct is; as we shall see, the size of the infarct can now be reduced by drugs called thrombolytics.

Heart attacks are common occurrences; in Britain alone, around quarter of a million people suffer a heart attack every year. Around two-thirds of them go on to make a full recovery. Half of all heart attack deaths occur within two hours of the onset of symptoms. The rest of the fatalities happen mainly in the year after the attack – often after the development of complications such as abnormal heart rhythms, heart failure, and valve problems – all of which can be treated by drugs.

A stroke occurs when the blood supply to the brain is interrupted. Around 80 per cent of strokes are due to a clot in one of the carotid arteries. The rest occur as a result of haemorrhage – when a blood vessel in the brain bursts, either through injury or because of congenital weakness. Around a quarter of all stroke victims die, another quarter recover completely and the rest are left with some degree of disability. Until very recently, there was no drug treatment available for stroke victims.

The heart's distress signal: angina

Angina is a symptom, not a disease. It is a gripping or crushing pain in the chest which occurs when the coronary arteries fail to supply the heart with enough oxygen for its needs. Angina is not the same as a heart attack; however, people with angina do run a three times greater risk of heart attack than the general population. The pain usually occurs on exertion, when the heart needs more oxygen than it does when at rest. If someone has narrowed arteries – usually because of atherosclerosis – the heart muscle will not receive enough oxygen-carrying blood to meet its demands. So it will 'cry out' in protest, producing anginal pain. On rest, the pain usually subsides (whereas the pain of a heart attack is not relieved by resting).

The faltering pump: heart failure

Heart failure is not always as serious as it sounds and should not be confused with cardiac arrest, which occurs when the heart actually stops beating. In heart failure, the output of blood from the heart to the rest of the body is not as high as it should be. This means that the other organs are not receiving the oxygen they need to function properly. Heart failure therefore puts a strain on the whole body.

The condition varies in its severity. People with mild heart failure can live fairly normal lives with the proper treatment. But advanced heart failure is a life-threatening condition. Heart failure is fairly common, and it is on the increase – mainly because of the general ageing of the population. Around three per cent of people over 65 have some degree of heart failure, and its overall incidence in the UK is about 0.4 per cent. The commonest cause of heart failure is myocardial infarction because of the failure of part of the heart's muscle that occurs in a heart attack. Other causes include high blood pressure (hypertension), mechanical defects such as heart valve disease, heart muscle disorders, and disorders of the heart rhythm. Sometimes the cause is not in the heart itself. In anaemia, for instance, there are fewer red blood cells than normal, so the oxygen carrying capacity of the blood is reduced. The heart's output needs to increase to compensate, and this may be above its normal maximum output.

When the heart's output drops a number of changes take place in the body. The heart ventricles enlarge. This causes an increase in the pressure of the blood inside them which is transmitted to the veins and capillaries throughout the body. It is more difficult for blood to enter the heart from the veins, so it starts to accumulate. The increased pressure causes fluid to seep from the blood vessels into the tissues, leading to congestion of the lungs and other organs. Doctors often talk of congestive heart failure, because of this 'waterlogging' of the tissues.

At the same time, the nervous system responds by increasing the rate and strength of the heart beat, and the kidneys start to conserve salt and water, aided by the release of powerful hormones. This further increases the blood pressure, worsening the congestion. Either the right or the left ventricle – or both – can fail.

Heart failure can lead to a number of complications. As the circulation becomes sluggish, clots in the leg veins become more likely; these become dangerous if they move round the body and lodge in the arteries serving the heart or brain. Lung congestion makes the patient very vulnerable to infection. And if they are deprived of oxygen for too long by a failing heart, the liver and kidneys will fail.

Heart failure is treatable with drugs; 90 per cent of people with mild heart failure will be able to live a normal life, given the right drugs. The outlook for patients with severe heart failure is not so good; half die within two years, either suddenly or from progression of the condition.

Hypertension: the silent killer

The force of blood being pumped through the arteries exerts pressure on their walls. This is commonly known as the blood pressure, and its value depends on the cardiac output, and the resistance that the artery walls offer to the flow of blood. Blood pressure has its maximum value, known as the systolic blood pressure, as the heart contracts. It then falls to a minimum value, the diastolic blood pressure, just before the next contraction. Doctors measure both systolic and diastolic blood pressures, so a blood pressure reading has two values. These are given in units called millimetres of mercury (mmHg). The values vary from person to person, and are affected by many other factors, but a typical value for a healthy young adult would be 120/80 (i.e. systolic pressure 120 mmHg, diastolic pressure 80 mmHg). Values tend to increase with age, at least in Western societies.

Blood pressure which is persistently greater than 140/90 in a person at rest is defined as hypertension (high blood pressure). It usually occurs when the arteries offer too much resistance to the flow of blood through them. Once the arterial resistance has increased, blood has to be forced through harder, creating increased pressure.

The majority of cases – about 90 per cent – are classified as essential hypertension, where there is no obvious underlying cause of the high blood pressure, although there are many theories. Abnormal sodium balance, for example, might lead to an increase in blood volume, which in turn raises the blood pressure. Or there may be high levels, or poor control, of hormones that constrict the blood vessels. There are probably several different, interacting, causes of essential hypertension.

The remaining ten per cent of patients with high blood pressure have secondary hypertension. Here there is an obvious reason for raised blood pressure. The commonest is taking the oral contraceptive pill. The risk of developing hypertension on the Pill is greatest in overweight women, long-term users (over five years) and in women over 35. Other causes of secondary hypertension include kidney disease and hormonal disorders such as Cushing's syndrome. It can be hard to separate cause and effect in the case of kidney disease, because hypertension can lead to kidney damage.

One per cent of patients suffer from a potentially fatal condition known as malignant hypertension in which there is a dramatic rise in the blood pressure to values around 200/140. Otherwise, hypertension is a chronic condition. It rarely gives rise to any symptoms and most people discover they have it only through a routine check. However, the stress on the arteries produced by hypertension can lead to long-term damage. Hypertension tends to produce atherosclerosis, which can lead to coronary heart disease, stroke and transient ischaemic attack (a temporary interruption of blood supply to the brain that often precedes a stroke). Hypertension is the major predisposing cause of cerebral haemorrhage, where weakened blood vessels in the brain burst. Kidney damage is another common complication of hypertension. And because the heart must work harder to push the blood through the narrowed arteries, left ventricular hypertrophy (the clinical term for an enlarged heart) followed by heart failure may occur.

Hypertension is probably responsible for 10 to 20 per cent of all deaths; it increases the risk of all cardiovascular disease two- to three-fold. Both drugs and lifestyle changes can lower blood pressure to normal levels and are therefore potentially life-saving. In the most recent study (discussed in more detail in the next section), there were 60 per cent fewer deaths among people whose hypertension was treated by drugs than among those who were not on drug therapy. So identification, monitoring, and treatment of patients with hypertension can reduce suffering and death from cardiovascular disease.

However, most people with hypertension feel perfectly well, so it requires a certain amount of commitment for them to keep their blood pressure under control, particularly if it involves taking drugs which may have side effects.

Assessing the risk factors in cardiovascular disease

Today most people have a pretty good idea of at least some of the things they can do to help avoid heart attacks and strokes – stop smoking, take exercise, eat a low-fat diet and so on. Prevention is especially important in CV disease. Around half of all deaths from coronary heart disease occur without any prior warning (you probably know of at least one such case), and only 20 per cent of heart attacks occur in people who already have angina. And most strokes are equally unexpected.

But 50 years ago, doctors thought that cardiovascular disease was just bad luck. And they frowned on the idea of offering patients advice when they had no symptoms; it was thought to be bad form to worry people unnecessarily.

The switch to preventative health care in CV disease came with some important epidemiological studies which were launched in the 1940s and 1950s. Epidemiology is the study of patterns of disease in the general population, and how these are shaped by the way people live. In a typical epidemiological project, researchers ask people questions about their lifestyle, covering areas such as diet, exercise, smoking habits and so on. They may also give them medical checks, monitoring blood pressure or hormone levels, for example. This data is collected over a period of time (the longer the better). The researchers will also monitor their subjects' health, looking at what diseases they suffer from and what they die of. They will then try to find links between the lifestyle factors and the illnesses that later develop. (Note that epidemiology is far wider in its scope than the clinical trials discussed in Chapter 3.) Most of the risk factors for common diseases have emerged from epidemiology – such as the link between smoking and lung cancer.

However, epidemiological studies do have a number of drawbacks. First, humans living freely are harder to control than humans in hospital undergoing, say, a clinical trial. They may give false information about their diet, for example, either because they forget or because they worry that the experimenter will disapprove of them if they admit to eating 15 Mars Bars in the previous week. Second, like a clinical trial, an epidemiological project must be well designed if the results are to have any meaning. To take a crude example, it is no good spending ten years researching the impact of carrot intake on lung cancer if you compare men who eat more than five carrots a day with women who eat fewer than three; if the women get more lung cancer, it might be due to their sex, rather than a lack of carrots. And finally, although epidemiology can make links between lifestyle and disease it cannot really show how a certain risk factor causes a disease. For that you need to supplement the epidemiology with laboratory experiments, usually on animals.

But good epidemiology has life-saving potential. Much of what we know about the risk factors for CV disease comes from the Framingham Heart Study. This giant epidemiological project started in 1948 in the small town of Framingham in Massachusetts and initially involved 5209 of its inhabitants. The Framingham researchers are now working with the children of the original volunteers. The work has produced hundreds of papers in the medical journals and is still turning up results of interest that affect the way doctors advise and prescribe. For instance, a recent report from Framingham showed that the risk of death from CV disease was 60 per cent lower among people on medication for hypertension than among people who were not taking drugs for the condition. This discovery is based on data collected for three different groups of men and women aged 50–59 over three different 20 year periods beginning in 1950, 1960 and 1970. So the whole study spans 40 years. It may affect the way doctors prescribe drugs for high blood pressure. Earlier studies of the benefits of these drugs have covered much shorter time periods, and have suggested that they are more useful in preventing stroke than heart attack. Now doctors may be more inclined to offer drug treatment for mild hypertension if they think they can help the patient cut the risk of heart attack as well as stroke.

Over the years epidemiology has shown the following lifestyle factors to be important in CV disease: smoking, diet, exercise and alcohol consumption. Smoking is a risk factor in its own right, while the other three can generate other CV disease risks such as obesity, hypertension, high cholesterol, and diabetes which can be hard to disentangle from one another. Lifestyle changes and medication can both decrease these risk factors. Increasingly, genetic factors are being recognised as having an impact on the risk of CV disease. These are not modifiable directly of course (at least, not yet) but people with a family history of CV disease have the most to gain from modifying their lifestyle to cut down on other risk factors.

Smoking: more than just lung cancer

Many doctors rate smoking as a greater risk factor for CV disease than either hypertension or obesity. Cigarette smoke appears to act as an irritant to the inner lining of the arteries, exacerbating atherosclerosis and increasing the risk of thrombosis. The risk increases with the number of cigarettes smoked. If you stop smoking, the risk decreases and after around ten years is thought to be similar to that of someone who has never smoked. The signs are that the smoking message has got through to people – at least in Western Europe and the United States, where the number of smokers has declined in recent years. This may be reflected in the falling rates of CV disease in these countries. However, smoking is on the increase in developing countries, particularly in China, and is still common in Eastern Europe and the former Soviet Union.

An apple a day – the impact of diet on CV disease

Eating habits play a major role in the incidence of coronary heart disease and stroke. It is widely recognised that a low fat, low salt, high carbohydrate diet, rich in fruit and vegetables, protects against CV disease.

In the UK, the Government's Committee on Medical Aspects of Food Policy (COMA) recommends cutting fat intake to 35 per cent of total calories (and only 11 per cent of the total should be from saturated fat). Fat and carbohydrate are the body's fuels and, when broken down during digestion, provide most of the energy (measured in Calories) in the daily diet. Fat is more energy dense than carbohydrate, providing 9 Calories per gram compared with 4 Calories per gram for carbohydrate. If 35 per cent of a typical daily diet of, say, 2000 Calories is to come from fat, then the fat has to provide only 700 Calories. At 9 Calories per gram, this represents a total fat intake of 78 g (of which only 24 g should be saturated fat). A corresponding increase of carbohydrate foods such as bread, rice and potatoes should make up the calorie deficit. A ten per cent reduction of saturated fat would lead to a reduction in mortality from coronary heart disease of 20–30 per cent, according to recent research.

Saturated fat increases the level of cholesterol – a component of plaque – in the blood. Fats, oils and cholesterol are all lipids, a large and diverse group of naturally occurring chemicals which are characterised by their insolubility in water. Fats, like butter and margarine, are solid at room temperature while oils are liquid. Both are composed of glycerol (or glycerine, as it is commonly known) chemically linked to substances called fatty acids; fats and oils are sometimes referred to as triglycerides because of this common chemical structure.

The type of fatty acid present in a fat or oil affects whether or not it is good for you. All fatty acid molecules contain carbon, hydrogen and oxygen atoms linked together according to the rules of chemical bonding. Saturated fatty acids contain carbon atoms which are bonded together in a different way from some of the carbon atoms in unsaturated fatty acids. A further distinction has to be made: monounsaturated fatty acids contain only two unsaturated carbon atoms, while polyunsaturated fatty acids contain more than two.

Hard margarine, dairy products, and meat are rich in saturated fatty acids, while vegetable oils are rich in unsaturated fatty acids. Saturated fatty acids raise blood cholesterol more than unsaturated fatty acids – hence the directive to keep down the amount of saturated fat.

Cholesterol is not all bad; it is an essential component of cell membranes, and several hormones are synthesised from it. The liver makes its own cholesterol, which is in addition to any dietary intake from food such as cream, milk, or eggs. Cholesterol is transported around the body in particles called lipoproteins in which the cholesterol is surrounded by a protein-rich coat. There are several types of lipoprotein, but for the purposes of this discussion we need only consider two. High density lipoprotein (HDL) carries excess cholesterol from the tissues to the liver, which will recycle it. It is commonly known as 'good' cholesterol. Low density lipoprotein (LDL), on the other hand, takes cholesterol that is stored in fat cells (the result of a high fat diet) and distributes it to other tissues, including the inner walls of the arteries.

Early research showed that people with coronary heart disease tend to have high blood cholesterol levels. In the late 1970s, it was shown that the distribution of this cholesterol between HDL and LDL is the really important factor. HDL decreases the risk of heart disease, while LDL increases it. So while a total blood cholesterol level of less than 5.2 millimoles per litre is desirable, the ratio of HDL to total blood cholesterol is more important.

Cholesterol levels can be lowered by diet, and by drugs. The main debate is over whether diets that lower cholesterol by a significant amount are palatable, and whether people will therefore be motivated to follow them long-term. You can replace saturated fats by unsaturated fats by adopting a Mediterranean style diet with an emphasis on fish and olive oil. Fish is rich in the so-called omega-3 polyunsaturated fatty acids and there is evidence that eating fatty fish like salmon or mackerel a couple of times a week will cut the risk of heart disease. Or you could replace the saturated fats with carbohydrates and opt for a rice-based Japanese style diet. On the available evidence, either diet is equally beneficial.

A diet which is less than ten per cent saturated fat – far below COMA's recommendations – lowers cholesterol by 10 per cent according to clinical studies. And one which has less than 7 per cent saturated fat will lower it by 20 per cent. This can bring high cholesterol into the normal range. The challenge to doctors and their coronary risk patients is whether such a diet can be made palatable and compatible with overall quality of life. Given that cholesterol can now be lowered effectively with drugs (discussed in the next section), an interesting debate is developing; take drugs long-term, risking side effects and long-term consequences, or develop self-discipline and motivation to achieve the same results through diet. Put like that it may sound as if the latter is the obvious 'moral' choice. Being realistic, however, the first option may turn out to be the most practical one for the people at risk of coronary heart disease.

There are also an increasing number of 'functional' foods coming onto the market which have either been processed to remove saturated fat and cholesterol, or which contain fat substitutes. In theory, these could help people reduce their saturated fat intake. However, sugar substitutes have been around for many years with the aim of helping people keep to a low-calorie diet and there is no evidence that they have made people either slimmer, or healthier. In addition, these foods pose a bit of a problem to the licensing authorities in some countries as they fall between two stools. They are, strictly, neither foods nor medicines. Manufacturers must beware making medical claims, or the product will have to go through the same testing and licensing programme as a pharmaceutical drug. Yet if specific claims are not made, it may be hard to market the foods. The same dilemma is faced by manufacturers of health foods and food supplements such as vitamins and minerals, and will be discussed in more detail in Chapter 10.

Apart from raising LDL and total cholesterol, the other major risk of a high fat diet is obesity. Overweight and obesity tend to be defined now in terms of body mass index (BMI) rather than just by weight alone. Your BMI can be calculated from dividing your weight in kilograms by the square of your height in metres. This should come up with a figure somewhere between 20 and 40. People with a BMI over 30 are classed as being obese. Anyone with a BMI between 25 and 30 is said to be overweight. Put another way, women with a waist measurement greater than 35 inches (40 inches for men) could benefit medically from losing weight.

People who are obese run a higher risk of coronary heart disease and stroke – mainly because they tend to have high blood pressure and an unfavourable lipid profile (high cholesterol and LDL, and low HDL). The majority of new cases of hypertension are attributable to overweight, especially in women. Weight loss can bring blood pressure down to normal levels without the need for medication. Obese people also often have insulin resistance and diabetes.

There are now several drugs being developed to treat obesity (of which more later) – but until such drugs have proved themselves and are generally available, dieting is the only realistic option. But it should be successful dieting; fluctuating weight – where someone diets, loses weight, then puts it back on – also seems to be risky. Less ambitious dieting – aiming to lose, say, just a few pounds rather than aim for an unrealistic target weight – is probably healthier in the long run. At the very least, obese people could usefully try not to put on any more weight. According to clinical studies, a 20 per cent weight loss in an obese person would give a 40 per cent reduction of coronary heart disease. And if everyone maintained their optimum weight (something you will have to work out for yourself, but somewhere around a BMI of 22) there would be a 25 per cent decrease in coronary heart disease and a 35 per cent fall in stroke and heart failure. The best way to do this is to tackle any modest weight gain (say between 5 and 10 pounds) right away.

Some heart specialists think that paying attention to the fruit and veg-etable component of diet will turn out to be even more important for cardio-vascular health than cutting down on saturated fat. The recommendation (at least in the UK, and few doctors elsewhere would disagree) is to eat five 80 gram helpings of fruit and vegetables a day. Fresh, tinned and frozen produce are fine, as are juices. But dried and pickled products do not count and nor do potatoes (which are classed as a carbohydrate).

This advice is based on several epidemiological studies which show that fruit and vegetables protect the cardiovascular system. In one study, 5000 Finnish men were rated on their fruit and vegetable consumption. The top third had a 34 per cent lower risk of a fatal heart attack than the bottom third. And a survey of 87,000 American nurses, carried out by JoAnn Manson of Brigham and Women's Hospital in Boston, reported a 26 per cent reduction in the risk of stroke among the fifth that ate most vegetables, compared with the fifth eating least.

The weak part of the fruit and vegetables argument is, of course, that people who eat a lot of fruit and vegetables may be healthier for other reasons; maybe they eat less fat, or exercise more, for example. And researchers are still not sure what substances in fruit and vegetables are important for cardiovascular protection. However, there is good evidence that they work by exerting an antioxidant effect on LDL, making it less damaging to the arteries.

Oxygen is essential to life, yet is is also a potent toxin. The second most reactive element on Earth, it attacks vital biological molecules within our cells with gusto – if left unchecked (more about this in Chapter 10). It hits on proteins, DNA and cell membranes causing damage which can lead to many cancers, many degenerative diseases (oxidative cell damage is thought to drive the ageing process) and heart disease. And LDL which has been oxidised is more likely than non-oxidised LDL to be incorporated into plaque.

There are natural antioxidants within our cells, such as the enzyme super-oxide dismutase. These intercept and deactivate oxygen before it can damage vital molecules within the cell. Boosting their levels with dietary antioxidants should be a good idea. The best-known antioxidants in fruit and vegetables are vitamins A, C and E. But more recently other substances with an antioxidant effect have been coming to the fore, such as polyphenols in red wine, and flavonoids in tea, apples and onions. Various studies have shown foods rich in all these nutrients to have a protective effect – particularly against stroke. For instance, Dutch scientists showed that the risk of heart attack was 49 per cent lower among men who ate 110 g or more apples a day (more than two decent-sized apples), compared with those who ate less than 18 g of apples a day.

If these antioxidants are so useful, why do companies not just make them

up into tablets, to save people the bother of calculating whether they have
eaten enough fruit and vegetables for the day? There are many supplements
on the market which aim to do just that. The most clinical research has been
done on vitamin E supplementation and the evidence for its effectiveness in
cardiovascular protection has been conflicting. Studies on beta-carotene (the
dietary precursor of vitamin A, and the substance that gives carrots their
orange colour) suggest that it is not useful, as a supplement, in protecting
against cardiovascular disease. The role of such supplements will be looked
at further in Chapter 10.

It has long been known that salt has an effect on blood pressure. Four
thousand years ago, Huang Li, the Yellow Emperor warned 'If too much
salt is used in food, the pulse hardens.' Most foods contain some salt, but
we only need about a teaspoon a day (and could probably get by on much
less). For every teaspoon over and above this, systolic blood pressure can
rise an extra 5–10 mmHg, which could be risky for someone whose blood
pressure is already too high.

There has been controversy too, over coffee. While it has been established
that the caffeine in coffee (see also Chapter 9) poses no special risk, there
are two substances in coffee beans – cafestol and kahweol – which can raise
cholesterol levels. These are removed by coffee filters, and do not occur to
a significant extent in instant or percolated coffee. However, boiled coffee,
which is popular in Scandinavia, Turkish coffee, and – as has recently been
shown – cafetière coffee have high enough levels of cafestol and kahweol to
have an adverse effect on cardiovascular risk if consumed in moderate to
high amounts (say six to eight strong cups of cafetière coffee a day).

Exercise and alcohol intake are the remaining two lifestyle factors which
are often discussed with respect to CV disease. Exercise has many benefits;
it counteracts the effects of stress hormones, which themselves may predispose to heart disease, lowers high blood pressure and keeps weight under
control. It also raises HDL levels.

Alcohol also reduces stress – at least when taken in moderation. There is
also mounting evidence that moderate intake can protect against heart disease. The protective effect starts at levels as low as one unit a day (a unit is
8 grams of alcohol – the equivalent to half a pint of average strength beer or
a small glass of wine), according to the most recent report by the UK'S
Department of Health. People who drink 7 to 40 units a week are thought
to be 30–50 per cent less likely to develop CHD compared to non-drinkers.
Alcohol raises HDL levels and also lowers LDL levels. It decreases the risk
of blood clots by making the blood less 'sticky'. Other mechanisms for the

protective effect are currently under investigation. And it looks increasingly likely that it is alcohol, rather than any other component of alcoholic drinks, which confers the benefits (it has long been assumed that something in red wine gave the French an advantage – they smoke a lot, but have low rates of heart disease).

Drugs to treat cardiovascular disease

Herbal medicines based on foxgloves had been used to treat heart failure for hundreds of years. In 1796, Birmingham physician William Withering extracted the active ingredient, digitalis, from one of these brews. Ahead of his time, Withering went on to do laboratory experiments and clinical trials which resulted in the development of digitalis as the first ever heart drug. Digoxin and digitoxin, the active compounds in Withering's foxglove extract, make the heart beat more forcefully, which helps the failing heart to deliver blood around the body. However, these two drugs are not much used today because they have a low therapeutic index (see Chapter 1). And doctors now have over 100 different medications to choose from for the treatment of heart failure, hypertension and other cardiovascular conditions; in the last 20 years or so there has been an explosion in the number of new drugs coming onto the market. Here we review the main categories of cardiovascular drugs.

Angiotensin converting enzyme (ACE) inhibitors

The angiotensin converting enzyme (ACE) inhibitors have been around since about 1981. There are eight drugs on the market of which captopril and enalapril are the most widely used. Several more are under development. They are used to treat hypertension, heart failure and after a heart attack.

ACE inhibitors work by interfering with a natural feedback mechanism for controlling blood pressure. When blood pressure falls beyond a normal value, the kidneys secrete an enzyme called renin. This converts an enzyme precursor called angiotensinogen into an active form called angiotensin I. This, in turn, is acted on by angiotensin converting enzyme (ACE) to produce angiotensin II. Experiments have shown that angiotensin II acts as a vasoconstrictor, and is the most powerful blood pressure increasing substance ever studied. But ACE has another function in the body. It catalyses the breakdown of bradykinin, a substance with many physiological functions including the triggering of pain and inflammation.

In 1965 Brazilian scientist Sérgio Ferreira was working on bradykinin when he discovered that an extract of the South American pit viper *Bothrops jararaca* could inhibit its breakdown. Later on, other researchers showed that an active ingredient of the snake extract also lowered blood pressure in animals. The effects on both bradykinin and blood pressure come from the inhibition of ACE. Unfortunately, the compound was not orally active – if patients were to benefit they would have to have injections, which is not a practical way of treating a chronic condition such as hypertension. Enter chemists at pharmaceutical company Squibb. They adapted the original ACE inhibitor to make an orally active drug, captopril.

There is a wealth of new clinical data on ACE inhibitors, but it appears to be taking doctors some time to catch up – the drugs are prescribed less than they might be. In hypertension, it is still common to start a patient off with a beta blocker or a diuretic and then switch to an ACE inhibitor if these do not work well. But increasingly, some doctors will prescribe an ACE inhibitor as the first line drug.

Many – but not all – clinical trials have shown that the ACE inhibitors work well in heart failure, increasing lifespan, and decreasing symptoms of breathlessness and fatigue. The main prescribing dilemma is how early to start treatment. Patients may develop a condition known as left ventricular dysfunction (LVD), a harbinger of heart failure, without any symptoms. The left ventricle is the chamber of the heart which pumps blood around the body. If weakened, by age or disease, it often malfunctions by pumping less blood than it should. ACE inhibitors may slow down – but do not reverse – LVD. In a big trial involving around 6000 patients, using ACE inhibitors early on did not have a significant effect on mortality but it did prevent the onset of clinical heart failure in 3 out of 100 patients treated. The latter result needs some explaining. Either these patients' symptoms were alleviated by the drug – so although their survival chances were not improved, at least their quality of life was better. Or the onset of disease really was being slowed down – in which case they would live longer. Further study of this type of response to ACE inhibitors is needed to find out what is really going on.

ACE inhibitors have also been used in patients who develop heart failure after a myocardial infarction. The most recent studies show that they save one life in every 85 patients treated.

Doctors usually start heart failure patients on ACE inhibitors under strict supervision in hospital. This is because these drugs sometimes cause a drastic fall in blood pressure which could be detrimental to patients who are already quite ill. By contrast, GPs can prescribe ACE inhibitors to patients with hypertension. In general, these patients feel well on ACE inhibitors – an important factor where treatment may well be lifelong. One side effect is a dry cough. This results from the irritant action of bradykinin in the lungs (ACE breaks down bradykinin, so ACE inhibitors keep its concentrations up). ACE inhibitors may cause problems with kidney function, which may be why some doctors are a little reluctant to prescribe them for patients with mild hypertension.

Calcium channel blockers

When the mineral calcium enters muscle cells, it triggers a whole cascade of biochemical responses whose outcome is contraction of the muscle. It enters through channels in specialised proteins which span the cell membrane. The calcium channels are just one example of a whole class of proteins known as ion channels that permit cells to make contact with their surroundings. They make possible two-way traffic of essential chemicals, like calcium, and waste products between the cell and its immediate surroundings.

Calcium channel blockers are drugs which bind to the channels and change their shape in such a way as to close the way through the membrane. They act upon smooth muscle, which lines the blood vessels, and on heart muscle. By cutting down on the amount of calcium entering the cell, the calcium channel blockers can affect the contraction of the heart and the tone of the blood vessels.

The three main calcium channel blockers used in CV disease are nifedipine, verapamil, and diltiazem – although there are around 20 more under development. Nifedipine has little effect upon the heart, but acts as a vasodilator and is so used in the treatment of hypertension. Doctors may prescribe it where beta blockers or diuretics are not suitable for a patient – but, like the ACE inhibitors, nifedipine is increasingly being used as the first line drug in high blood pressure. Verapamil and diltiazem act mainly on heart muscle and are used mainly in the treatment of angina. By reducing the force of the muscle contraction of the heart, they allow it to ease up on its workload and oxygen demand.

Clinical trials to assess the use of verapamil and diltiazem in heart failure and after myocardial infarction are underway. The first indications are that they do improve prognosis if used with caution in carefully selected patient groups.

Common side effects with nifedipine include dizziness and flushing – in fact, just what you would expect from a potent vasodilator. Verapamil is usually very well tolerated, except that it may produce constipation because it decreases contraction of the smooth muscle of the gastrointestinal tract, and the passage of its contents is therefore slowed down.

Beta blockers

The autonomic nervous system (ANS) controls many bodily functions, including circulation. The ANS works on a negative feedback principle (as was also discussed in the previous chapter); information from various parts of the body is processed in the hypothalamus and medulla, both control centres of the brain. To make the appropriate adjustment in bodily function (e.g. to speed up a heart that is not beating hard enough), electrical impulses pass down the nerves towards the relevant organ. This results in the release of neurotransmitter substances, which act upon the cells of the organ, producing an appropriate physiological adjustment.

The ANS is divided, on anatomical grounds, into two branches – sympathetic and parasympathetic. Some parts of the body, such as the heart, gut wall and salivary glands, are acted on by both branches. In general, the two branches of the ANS have opposing effects. The activity of the sympathetic nervous system, through its neurotransmitter substance noradrenaline, leads to a 'flight or fright' response to danger. Noradrenaline is also secreted as a hormone from the adrenal gland, along with its close relative adrenaline (see Chapter 4) with similar effects.

Dilated pupils, widening of the air tubes in the lungs, and increased heart rate are all the result of noradrenaline or adrenaline acting on specific receptors on the organ involved. This is where drugs come in; there are three different types of adrenoreceptor – α, β_1 and β_2. An organ may have more than one type of receptor. For instance, blood vessels have both α and β_2 receptors. Alpha receptors tend to be more responsive to noradrenaline, while beta receptors respond more readily to adrenaline. The resulting physiological response depends upon which receptor is activated. Activation of alpha receptors on blood vessels leads to their constriction, while activation of beta receptors gives vasodilation, the opposite effect. Drugs which

bind selectively to adrenoreceptors have great potential to modify physiological responses.

And so to the beta blockers. Beta$_1$ blockers, such as atenolol, bind to
receptors in the heart, blocking the approach of noradrenaline and so slowing heart rate (where noradrenaline would increase it). Atenolol and related
drugs are very widely used in the treatment of hypertension and angina.
Lowering the heart rate decreases the stress on the blood vessels and therefore reduces blood pressure. Beta blockers are often used to reduce the
physical symptoms of anxiety such as palpitations, shaking hands, sweating
and over-breathing. Musicians, and dart-players, often take beta blockers
to steady their hand, and they are widely prescribed for stage fright.

They have also been tried after myocardial infarction where a single
dose appears to reduce the area of damaged muscle as well as stabilising
ventricular fibrillation (a condition in which the ventricles of the heart beat
in an unco-ordinated and useless way). Used on a regular basis in the year
following a heart attack, beta blockers appear to reduce mortality. Their use
in heart failure is controversial; some studies show they make heart failure
worse, while more recent trials, using newer drugs such as carvedilol, show
an opposite result.

Beta$_1$ receptors are found in the heart and intestinal smooth muscle, while
β_2 receptors occur in bronchial muscle and in the blood vessels. If the beta
blocker is not sufficiently selective for the heart's β_1 receptors it will have
marked side effects. For instance, asthma may be made worse by broncho-
spasm, as adrenaline normally dilates the airways. Cold hands and feet are
very common on beta blockers, for reasons which are not fully understood.
It appears that they mimic the vasoconstricting effect of noradrenaline on
the peripheral blood vessels.

Diuretics

For many years, diuretics have been the mainstay of the treatment of both
hypertension and heart failure. They act on the kidneys, increasing their
output of urine. This decreases the tension in the blood vessels. It also
reduces the waterlogging (swollen ankles and fluid in the lungs) which is
typical of heart failure. There are three kinds of diuretic drug in common
use: thiazides, loop, and potassium-sparing. They all work at slightly different places in the kidney, and basically stop it reabsorbing water and sodium
chloride.

Thiazide diuretics such as bendrofluazide have a relatively weak action; clinical trials show they decrease the incidence of stroke. Frusemide, used mainly for heart failure, is a loop diuretic and is more potent than a thiazide diuretic. Finally, the potassium-sparing diuretics such as amiloride protect the body from loss of the vital mineral potassium. On a diuretic, the body loses potassium along with the extra water. While this can be replaced by including plenty of potassium-rich foods such as dried apricots and bananas, some patients may be especially vulnerable to potassium loss and therefore would benefit from these drugs.

Aspirin again

Aspirin had been in use as a painkiller and anti-inflammatory before its potential application in CV disease was suspected. As was discussed in Chapter 1, the enzyme cyclooxygenase (COX) turns arachidonic acid into hormones called prostaglandins. These contribute to pain and inflammation at the site of an injury. However, in the endothelial cells which line blood vessels, prostaglandins are transformed into prostacyclin, a potent vaso-dilator. But in blood platelets, the prostaglandins are turned, instead, into a substance called thromboxane, which actually constricts the blood vessels, as well as inducing platelets to aggregate to form a clot. You might think therefore that the effects of aspirin in the blood vessels would cancel out.

In fact, it has long been known that aspirin has an overall thinning effect upon the blood; this is one of its commonest side effects. People who are especially sensitive to aspirin may suffer excess bleeding after dental sur-gery, or injury, if they take it long-term. What appears to happen is that the COX in the endothelial cells is only affected for a short time by aspirin. New COX molecules are produced, leaving prostacyclin production largely unaffected. However, platelets cannot make more COX and so the effect of aspirin on them is permanent, so long as the dose is kept up.

Around 75–100 mg aspirin a day (half a regular aspirin) appears to be effective in a number of cardiovascular conditions. In 1994, major clinical trials were published in Britain which suggested that regular aspirin could save one hundred thousand premature deaths a year, worldwide, from stroke or heart attack. In addition, many more non-fatal, but disabling, cardiovas-cular events would be prevented. In one trial, the occurrence of death, non-fatal stroke or non-fatal heart attack in a group was reduced to ten per cent, compared to 14 per cent in the control group, in three types of patient –

those with suspected acute heart attack, and those who had a previous heart attack or stroke. Similar results were found in patients with angina and blood clots in the leg. Aspirin also protected people undergoing bypass surgery or angioplasty to unblock coronary arteries from occurrence of clots (a common complication of such surgery). In addition, aspirin cuts the incidence of stroke among patients who have suffered a transient ischaemic attack (TIA). In TIA, the blood supply to the brain is briefly interrupted – a sure sign of narrowed cerebral arteries and therefore a warning sign of a future stroke. And it is also useful in treatment of pregnancy-induced hypertension (pre-eclampsia) which is potentially fatal to both mother and baby.

Further studies are being undertaken, to ascertain whether aspirin is also useful for people with hypertension, diabetes, high cholesterol or for smokers – that is, people with isolated risk factors. In the United States, recommendations have just been broadened to include patients with angina, and others at high risk of a first heart attack (in other words, there is now a shift towards primary prevention). Aspirin is also used in first aid when there is a strong suspicion of heart attack and with stroke if the medical personnel are pretty sure the stroke is caused by a blocked vessel (85 per cent of strokes are of this kind, but the rest are caused by bleeding into the brain and aspirin will make these worse). In the biggest ever trial of stroke treatment, reported recently, aspirin was shown to be beneficial to stroke patients if given within three hours of the event and continued indefinitely. This time window allows time for scans to show if the stroke is indeed from a clot (aspirin will be of no use in haemorrhagic stroke). If a million patients are treated with aspirin in this way, 10,000 will be saved from a second stroke while they are in hospital.

Incidentally, aspirin has also been shown to protect against Alzheimer's disease and some forms of cancer. But you still shouldn't self-prescribe it (although many doctors admit they take it themselves) just in case you are one of the few people who are sensitive to its side effects. However, this recommendation may change as further research is reported.

Statins – keeping cholesterol at bay

The statins are cholesterol-lowering drugs. Fairly new on the market, they are already being used widely in people with cholesterol levels over 6.5 mmol/L. Ideally, these people will have tried a low-fat diet first to get their cholesterol within normal limits. Statins are inhibitors of the enzyme hydroxymethylglutaryl coenzyme A, which is involved in the production of the body's natural cholesterol in the liver.

The four statins on the market are simvastatin, pravastatin, lovastatin and – most recently – atorvastatin. They all appear to be well tolerated and effective. There have been a number of big clinical trials on the protective effects of statins, and more are underway. For instance the so-called 4S trial (Scandinavian Simvastatin Survival Study) has enrolled 5000 people with coronary heart disease and cholesterol between 5.5 and 8 mmol/L. Interim results show a decrease in total cholesterol of 25 per cent. Low density cholesterol was down by 35 per cent, and HDL was up by 8 per cent. As far as mortality is concerned, 12 per cent of the placebo group died, compared to 8 per cent in the simvastatin group, while 28 per cent of the placebo group had heart attacks compared to 19 per cent in the treatment group.

Even more promising are results from an ongoing trial of Scottish men with high cholesterol, but without coronary heart disease. Pravastatin reduced the incidence of heart attack in these men by a third. Other studies have tended to confirm these results.

The main drawback of statins is that there is some evidence that overall mortality, particularly from accidental death, suicide and murder, appears to be increased. Not all studies have shown this, however.

Based on the data so far, if everyone who could benefit in the UK took statins, there would be 1910 fewer deaths from CHD, and less morbidity and medical costs from heart attacks. But the drugs would cost around £200 million per annum and it would take several years for savings to show up in terms of healthcare costs.

Drugs for obesity – an impossible dream?

Diet drugs, in the future, may turn out to be rather like the statins – giving people a helping hand with lifestyle changes that could reduce their overall risk of CV disease. Obesity has been difficult to treat and not just because of problems with the drugs used to help people lose weight (discussed below). The trouble is that until recently, doctors have tended to view excess weight as a failure of willpower on the part of the patient, rather than as a genuine clinical condition. This may be changing – the emerging view is that some people *are* genetically predisposed to weight gain.

Look at the Pima Indians. If they migrate to Arizona, they have a 70 per cent rate of obesity, while in their native Mexico, where they stick to a traditional lifestyle, they are no fatter than anyone else. Genes that help people squirrel away food, in a physiological sense, in times of scarcity have great survival value – but do not serve us well in times of plenty. It may be that some populations, like the Pima Indians, bear especially efficient versions of such genes. So they may have been able to survive for longer than other people on a kill in hunter-gatherer days. Nowadays, when they eat hamburgers and chips, they have become the people who just cannot burn off the calories. There is much research still to be done. But it may be there is more truth to the excuse 'It's my genes, Doctor,' than there ever was in the plaintive 'It's my glands, Doctor.'

The other problem with obesity is that the condition is also bound up with image – most people like to look slim. People with high cholesterol levels or hypertension do not worry about what they look like (unless they are also overweight, of course) and do not expect their medicine to make them look more attractive. But there are millions of overweight people, who are not clinically obese, who would be happy to take diet drugs just to improve their image by shedding a few pounds. Diet drugs are – and always have been – open to misuse by healthy people.

The facts about weight control are simple enough (even though the underlying biochemical and physiological mechanisms are not). The body needs to balance calorie intake (food and drink) with calorie output (activity and exercise). Any imbalance is stored as fat. To keep the intake–output equation in balance, you have to cut calories and increase energy output – in other words, resist any tendency to gluttony or sloth (most doctors reckon not taking enough exercise is what lies at the bottom of most weight problems). Any diet drug that's going to work has to do the same thing. Either it has to reduce food intake, or burn it off more efficiently – simulating the effect of vigorous exercise.

The first drugs to be used for weight control were the amphetamines in the 1930s. These stimulants decrease appetite by acting on the hypothalamus, the part of the brain that controls food intake. But amphetamines have serious side effects such as raised blood pressure and palpitations. Long-term use leads to dependence, and they can be fatal in overdose. So most doctors stopped prescribing them in the 1960s – although they may still be on offer at private slimming clinics.

Amphetamines have been replaced by a group of similar, but less harmful drugs. Two which are often used are diethylpropion (trade names: Tenuate, Dospan and Apesate), and phentermine (Duromine, Ionamin). These are also stimulants that increase levels of the brain chemical noradrenaline. This decreases appetite, but also hypes you up – leading to side effects that include restlessness, dry throat and insomnia.

The problem is that the drugs don't really work that well. Tests on phentermine show that it gives a weight loss of half a pound a week for about a month. Stop taking it and the weight piles back on. Another drug, fenfluramine (Ponderax), acts differently; it boosts levels of another brain chemical, serotonin, and makes you feel full. The anti-depressant Prozac also works on serotonin (see also Chapter 8), but unfortunately only produces weight loss at very high doses. Side effects of fenfluramine include drowsiness and diarrhoea – but it's less likely to be addictive than the stimulating drugs.

However, fenfluramine and a drug closely related in structure, dexfenfluramine (Adifax), have just been withdrawn from the market. A US study of 291 patients on these drugs showed a 30 per cent rate of heart valve defects. These would not necessarily give rise to symptoms, but could progress over time to potentially fatal cardiac weaknesses. Dexfenfluramine also carries a slight risk of pulmonary hypertension, a dangerous form of high blood pressure affecting the lungs, and has been shown to cause brain damage in animals.

Opinion is divided on the value of these two drugs – and how big a setback their withdrawal will be. Trials showed only a modest weight loss of about half a stone (3 kg) over three months for patients on dexfenfluramine. But a combination of fenfluramine and phentermine known as sibutramine (trade name Reductil) gives more impressive results; of 4000 failed dieters who tried the drug, nine out of ten lost a stone (6.3 kg) and kept it off for over a year. For the severely obese, even this modest weight loss could provide health benefits and provide motivation for long-term weight control. But for the merely overweight, the risks of these drugs are greater than the potential benefit. Under the new rules sibutramine will not be available, because of its fenfluramine component.

However, there are other ways of attacking the intake–output weight equation. Another way of cutting food intake is to bulk up food with substances that won't be absorbed by the body. Bulking agents like methylcellulose (Celevac) make you feel full, but also give rise to flatulence, bloating and even intestinal obstruction. Then there are drugs like acarbose, available on prescription in Europe, which stops the body from breaking down carbohydrate. Unfortunately, acarbose doesn't lead to any significant weight loss (it is really meant to control blood sugar) and leads to flatulence from fermentation of undigested carbohydrate. Under development is orlistat, which stops the digestion of fat; you can eat fatty foods, but they will pass straight through the body.

And then there are drugs to tackle the other side of the weight control equation by burning off food more efficiently – mimicking the effect of a jog or an aerobics class. The first of these so–called thermogenic drugs was discovered by accident during the first World War. Munitions workers handling the explosives ingredient dinitrophenol (DNP) reported sweating and weight loss. DNP was promoted for a while as a slimming drug, but it was found to be very toxic and led to a number of deaths. There are many other drugs that speed up the rate of food burning – even alcohol and caffeine – although the effects are short-lived. A doctor in Denmark noticed that asthmatics given a drug containing ephedrine lost weight, and a prep-aration containing ephedrine and caffeine is now marketed as a thermogenic drug in Denmark (although ephedrine – a component of 'herbal' Ecstasy and some traditional Chinese herbal remedies – has been associated with several deaths and cannot be recommended – see also Chapter 10). Many drug companies are still working on more sophisticated, and safer, versions of thermogenic drugs, but the problem to date has been ironing out the side effects.

The big breakthrough that promises a new era in hi-tech anti-fat drugs came in 1994 when Jeffrey Friedman of the Rockefeller Institute in New York announced that mice with mutations in a gene called 'ob' could not stop eating. They became massively fat – weighing three times as much as their normal counterparts. The ob gene operates in fat cells and produces a hormone called leptin that sends a message to the hypothalamus which says that fat stores are sufficient. This should stop the mice eating, at least temporarily. When there is no leptin present – because the mutated ob gene cannot produce any – the mice just carry on feeding.

Excitement mounted when further experiments showed that injections of leptin normalised the weight of the obese mice. Shares in Amgen, the biotechnology giant which spent $90 million on the rights to develop leptin for humans, leapt in value overnight. No one has shown that mutations in the human equivalent of the ob gene lead to obesity. In fact obese people have normal or even high leptin levels. Recent discoveries suggest that these people may have a defective leptin receptor in the hypothalamus – in other words, the leptin message is just not getting through.

And there could be spin-off drugs from leptin. When leptin acts on the hypothalamus, it turns off production of a chemical called neuropeptide Y

(NPY) which is a powerful feeding stimulant. Drugs that act as antagonists to NPY could reduce appetite. It has also been shown that if the so-called melanocortin 4 receptor in the hypothalamus is stimulated animals eat less. Therefore agonist drugs to this receptor could also reduce appetite and many companies are now working on this target.

Another class of drug under development for obesity aims to mimic the chemical signals which the stomach sends to the brain when it is full. One is glucagon-like peptide (GLP-1) discovered by Steve Bloom, at Hammersmith Hospital in London. GLP-1 is produced by rats after eating and acts as a chemical messenger saying the stomach is full. If GLP-1 is blocked by other chemicals, mice overeat. And there is also cholecystokinin (CCK), a hormone produced by the digestive system which acts similarly to GLP-1. Some doctors believe that people who binge eat may have some defect in CCK production and maybe a CCK-like drug could help them normalise their eating patterns.

And finally, there are β_3 adrenoreceptors on fat cells which enable the release of fat into the blood and burn it as fuel. As you might expect, these are part and parcel of the adrenaline response to stress and help supply the body with extra energy. In the context of weight control, agonist drugs – currently in preclinical development – could help balance the intake/ouput equation by burning off calories.

There are bound to be more drugs in the anti-obesity pipeline in the next few years, for researchers reckoned that there are at least 30 different genes involved in the control of appetite and weight.

Thrombolytics

Thrombolytic drugs are designed for use in an emergency to dissolve a life-threatening clot in the vessels leading to the heart or brain. Normally, when a clot forms, an enzyme called plasmin eventually breaks it down. Clots are made of platelets trapped in a mesh of a thread-like protein called fibrin. Plasmin breaks down fibrin. It normally exists in the body in an inactive form called plasminogen (otherwise clots would break down before they could seal a wound). Plasminogen is activated via another enzyme called tissue plasminogen activator during clotting. Thrombolytics are drugs which can activate plasmin. There are four main thrombolytics in use: streptokinase, urokinase, alteplase and anistreplase.

Streptokinase is extracted from bacteria called haemolytic streptococci.

It can dissolve the clot, restoring the flow of blood to the heart in four out of five patients. Large clinical trials show that it decreases mortality from heart attack by around 21 per cent. And the sooner treatment is initiated the better. Ideally, all thrombolytics should be given less than four hours after the onset of heart attack pain – but treatment can be delayed up to 24 hours and there will still be some benefit in terms of survival.

Any drugs which are to be administed by paramedics or GPs rather than by hospital staff should be easy to administer. Urokinase, which is isolated from human urine, can be given as a simple injection while streptokinase has to be given as a drip infusion over an hour. You can imagine which one a busy doctor would prefer. Unfortunately, while streptokinase and urokinase are about equally effective in opening up blocked arteries, urokinase is far more expensive. It has also been the subject of fewer clinical studies than other thrombolytics, which rather undermines doctors' confidence in using it.

Recombinant tissue plasminogen activator (rtPA) is like the body's own plasminogen activator but has been made by genetic engineering (for more on genetically engineered drugs see Chapter 11). It has the advantage of having a local action for it only binds to plasminogen which is already attached to the fibrin of the clot. This is important; urokinase and streptokinase act on plasminogen everywhere in the circulation and so can cause unwanted bleeding by impairing the body's natural clotting ability. Recombinant tPA reduces mortality from heart attack by 26 per cent when compared with placebo.

Anistreplase (APSAC) is a chemically modified version of rtPA which is only broken down to its active form when it reaches the clot. It showed a 47 per cent reduction in heart attack mortality against placebo.

Cost of these four drugs varies. Steptokinase is cheapest at around £80 a shot, while corresponding treatments with urokinase, rtPA and APSAC cost £460, £750 and £495 respectively. In early trials no mortality difference was shown between streptokinase, rtPA and APSAC. However, if rtPA is given as a rapid infusion along with the anticoagulant heparin, there is a 14 per cent reduction in mortality over streptokinase.

Pre-hospital thrombolysis is said to save one life in ten for heart attack while the risk of a stroke (from unwanted bleeding) is 1 in 1000. Thrombolysis has recently been approved as a treatment for stroke. This is a real breakthrough; stroke has never until now been seen as an emergency – even though it is as serious as a heart attack – because there has been no real treatment. However, if rtPA is given within three hours of the stroke (allowing time to establish the cause of the stroke, as with aspirin) 31 per cent of patients will suffer no subsequent disability compared to only 20 per cent of those not given thrombolytics.

When the oxygen supply to the brain is cut off because of a clot, extensive damage to neurons occurs. This is the cause of the disability – loss of speech or paralysis – which often follows a stroke. Neurons traumatised by lack of oxygen act in a strange way. They often pump out a messenger chemical called glutamate (further discussed in Chapter 8) which in turn causes calcium ions to rush into the cells. This activates enzymes which destroy cell membranes and eventually leads to a form of biochemical mayhem known as excitotoxic cell death. Drugs such as Cerestat, which is being developed by Cambridge NeuroScience in Massachusetts, aim to block the action of glutamate and so protect the threatened neurons.

The pharmaceutical industry has responded impressively to the challenge of CV disease. The array of drugs on offer tackle the problem at every stage. Statins and anti-obesity drugs may be able to help people minimise the risk of developing heart disease. There are effective drugs to alleviate chronic conditions like hypertension and angina. And now there are drugs which can save lives in CV emergencies.

However, many of these drugs are quite new. Only time will tell what their impact on cardiovascular disease will be. One thing is certain, they will never be enough, on their own, to defeat the biggest killer in the Western world. They can only work alongside sensible lifestyle choices.

Cardiovascular disease is very much a modern problem. In the next chapter we will look at how drugs can help relieve the oldest medical problem in the world – pain.

6

The problem of pain

The experience of pain is almost universal. There are perhaps 100 people in the world who have been born with a genetic defect which leaves them unable to feel pain. They have to learn to make their way through life without any natural protection from serious injury. For the rest of us pain is a sign that something is wrong. Painkillers, or analgesics, which are the most widely used of all drugs, may get rid of the pain, although they will not tackle the underlying cause. Thanks to drugs like aspirin and morphine, hardly anyone today need fear the misery of pain. But effective relief relies on matching the drug to the pain – which is sometimes a considerable challenge.

Understanding pain

Even the experts have difficulty in pinning down just what pain is. According to the International Association for the Study of Pain, it is an unpleasant sensory and emotional experience associated with actual or potential tissue damage. There are no blood tests, scans, or other laboratory measures which can diagnose pain. Where pain is a clinical problem, doctors rely on the patient describing their pain via a questionnaire. One of the most widely used tests, the McGill Pain Questionnaire, uses up to one hundred words – from 'gnawing' or 'piercing' to 'pounding' or 'shooting' – to try to capture the patient's experience.

The perception of pain goes far beyond its physical cause. It also depends upon cultural background, psychological experience, and the patient's current situation. Individual variations in pain experience have been assessed by measuring lower and upper pain thresholds under laboratory conditions. The lower pain threshold is the minimum intensity of painful stimulus – such as electric shock, pinprick, heat or pressure – perceived as painful. The upper threshold, or tolerance, is the intensity at which the volunteer will ask for the stimulus to be stopped. Experiments showed that levels of heat perceived as painful by Mediterranean people were experienced as warmth by Northern Europeans. But the most striking cultural and ethnic differences are in pain tolerance. For instance, women of Italian origin are less tolerant of pain than women of Old American or Jewish origin – at least in laboratory experiments. And many people, regardless of origin, can apparently ignore the pain of a heart attack. Electrocardiograms show that the damage suffered by people who have had 'silent' heart attacks is no less than those who experience crushing chest pain, which many describe as the worst of their life.

The way you experience pain may also depend on your previous experience. If your parents encouraged stoicism, then you may not seek help for pain as an adult. And the way pain is perceived may depend on what else is happening. If you learn that a friend has stomach cancer, a mild stomach cramp may be experienced as severe pain. Conversely, good news or excitement may lower the intensity of pain, or even make it disappear. Look at the way footballers often play on after injury, unaware of their pain until the game is over.

The way brain and body interact to produce such a wide spectrum of pain experience has preoccupied researchers since the 17th century. The great French philosopher René Descartes (1596–1650) likened the pain system to the bell-ringing mechanism in a church. Pain signals from the skin, when it is cut or burned, are like a man pulling on a rope at the bottom of the tower. The rope is a simple path the signals take through the body, reaching the brain, which is like the belfry. When the signals reach the brain, they set off a warning like a bell – and pain is perceived.

Of course, the physiology of pain turns out to be much more complicated than this; even now it is not fully understood. Scattered around the body are free nerve endings called nociceptors which respond to stimuli such as pressure, heat, electric shock, and chemicals released from nearby cells in response to injury. Nociceptors are present in most parts of the body, apart from brain tissue which does not have any. Tissues vary in their sensitivity to pain. A needle in the skin is more painful than one in a muscle. Cutting the intestines does not hurt (but you need an anaesthetic for abdominal surgery because the surgeon cuts through skin and muscle) but stretching or contracting them does.

Pain stimuli picked up by nociceptors pass along nerve fibres into the spinal cord. They are ferried through a vertical column of neurons called the dorsal horn to the thalamus, the brain's control centre, which is situated deep inside the skull, towards the back of the head. From here, signals spread out to other brain areas, such as the limbic system which is concerned with emotional response. It is incorrect to say there is a pain centre in the brain – although this was believed for many years.

Sometimes pain will be perceived as coming from a site of the body other than its real origin. This is known as referred pain. The pain of a heart attack is often felt in the left shoulder, arm or hand. Why this happens is not fully understood, but it may be because nerves from both regions (in this example the heart and the left arm) feel into a common pool of neurons in the dorsal horn. Therefore their origins could be confused by the brain when it receives the pain message.

Today, most physiologists accept the gate theory of pain put forward by Ronald Melzack and Patrick Wall in 1965. Put simply, this theory states that perception of pain can be modified at the level of the spinal cord – particularly by messages coming from the brain itself. The discovery of receptors for opiate painkillers, such as morphine, in the spinal cord lent support to the theory. These drugs can block pain messages from ascending to the brain. The theory also led to the development of spinal, or epidural, analgesia in which painkilling drugs are injected within the spinal cord.

There are various classifications of pain which may guide the choice of painkiller. Acute pain is the immediate response to injury, and results in a reflex action which causes you to withdraw from the threat. This pain is brief, sharp, and may be replaced by pain of a dull, throbbing nature after the injury. Toothache, period pain, and headache also fall into this category – although these everyday pains do not really produce a reflex response. A second category is reparative pain, which protects the body from further injury. Post-operative pain, or pain from a broken limb, forces you to rest so that the injury can heal. The pain in these two categories has an obvious protective function.

Those few people who cannot feel pain, mentioned above, are at risk throughout their lives. The best-documented case was the daughter of a Canadian doctor who soon developed severe problems with her knees, hips and spine. Because she never felt even the slightest pain on everyday injuries, she carried on regardless, so that the damage to her overworked joints never had a chance to heal. Injured tissue is particularly prone to invasion by bacteria. and this young woman died, aged 29, from massive infection.

But there is a third category of pain, known as chronic pain, which appears to have no function. In chronic pain, there is no obvious link between cause and effect – for instance, in arthritis, the extent of joint inflammation does not always correlate with the intensity of pain experienced. Chronic pain affects two per cent of the population and is a serious clinical condition which is often difficult to treat.

However, there is hope in sight because recent experiments on animals have provided new insights into the mechanisms of chronic pain. If the sciatic nerve, in the leg, was damaged in rats, the nervous system appeared to rewire itself in response. The main feature of the rewiring was the appearance of new nerve fibres in the dorsal horn, which could contact neurons that relay pain messages to the brain. Under these conditions, pain could be felt in response to non-pain stimuli, such as touch or vibration. The rat injuries simulate the circumstances under which intractable, chronic pain develops in humans. The new nerves probably grow under the influence of a natural chemical called nerve growth factor (NGF). Certainly, mice genetically modified to produce more NGF than normal do show extreme sensitivity to pain.

Pain in practice

There are many types of clinical pain for which analgesics might be prescribed. Here we will look at three of the most important types of pain: headaches, arthritis, and cancer pain.

The International Headache Society defines no fewer than 100 different types of headache. Curiously, the commonest headache – which we will call tension headache – is the least well understood. Four out of five people suffer tension headache. It is commonly assumed that this headache is triggered by contraction of muscles in the neck and the base of the skull. The resulting tension supposedly affects nerves in the scalp and produces a dull, aching, throbbing pain, perhaps accompanied by the sensation of having a tight band around the head. However, muscle tension is not always detectable in people with the symptoms of tension headache. And even when it is present, experts disagree as to whether the tension is the cause, or the effect, of the headache.

An acute tension headache rarely sends anyone to the doctor. A simple analgesic, like aspirin or paracetamol, rest, and avoidance of the trigger of the headache – such as a stuffy room, or glaring lights – are usually effective in relieving the pain. It is when it becomes chronic that tension headache becomes a real problem. Sometimes problems with the teeth, jaw, or neck are responsible for tension headache, and a visit to the dentist or physiotherapist may clear it up. Problems with the brain itself are never the cause – although worrying that you have a brain tumour will probably make your headache worse.

The majority of people with chronic headache show symptoms of depression; though it is not obvious whether this is the cause or the effect of the headache. Whatever the underlying cause, painkillers are not usually the answer. Indeed, patients with headaches that go on for months have often compounded the problem by becoming dependent on a daily dose of painkiller and perhaps caffeine as well. The chronic headache often responds instead to anti-depressant drugs, such as amitriptyline, or to non-drug therapy such as biofeedback, relaxation, or psychotherapy.

Migraine is far more dramatic than tension headache and affects an estimated 10 per cent of the population. An attack is often preceded by visual disturbances such as spots before the eyes, transient blindness and flashes of light, and feelings of dread – or euphoria – together with nausea and perhaps weakness, clumsiness and lack of co-ordination. The headache, when it arrives, can be devastating; the sufferer may have to lie prostrated in a darkened room for several hours or even for a day or so. The causes of migraine are not well understood, but it is a vascular headache, originating in contraction and then dilation of blood vessels in the brain, brought about by certain triggers. The neurotransmitter serotonin is thought to play a role, possibly by causing the blood vessels to dilate.

The neurological symptoms that usher in the headache are associated with the contraction phase, when the oxygen supply to the brain is diminished. When the blood vessels dilate, this probably impacts on nearby cranial nerves producing pain. Common triggers for migraine include chocolate, cheese, and the contraceptive pill. Ordinary painkillers, like aspirin or paracetamol, may help if taken in the early stages of an attack. Otherwise there is a newish drug called sumatriptan which resembles serotonin and may modify its action on the blood vessels. There is also a herbal remedy, feverfew, which has been shown to be effective in relieving migraine.

Arthritis is a common disease characterised by inflammation of the joints, which causes pain and swelling. There are several forms of arthritis, which together affect around one person in three. Osteoarthritis results from wear and tear on the joints. The protective cartilage tissue which covers the ends of the two bones in a joint breaks down, leaving the bare bones to contact one another and perhaps fragment, causing inflammation and pain. In rheumatoid arthritis, there is usually very obvious pain, swelling, joint deformity and perhaps even fever. Rheumatoid arthritis affects more women than men and typically sets in at a younger age than osteoarthritis. It may also affect the internal organs of the body, as well as the joints. Neither form of arthritis is curable; however, if it is caught early enough most sufferers can lead a reasonably normal life. The first line drugs used in relieving the symptoms of arthritis are the non-steroidal anti-inflammatory drugs (NSAID, discussed in more detail below).

Cancer affects one person in three at some time in their life (see the next chapter) and pain is perhaps the most dreaded symptom of the disease. It is estimated that around 70 per cent of all patients with advanced cancer suffer pain – which can be very severe. Most cancer pain arises from the tumour invading neighbouring tissue – the rest comes from cancer therapies. The nature of the pain depends upon where the cancer is. Dull, aching pain can come from tumours which have spread to the bone. Cancers which spread to the liver cause cramping abdominal pain. And if a tumour presses directly on a nerve, it may cause a sharp pain.

If unrelieved, pain can seriously affect the cancer patient's physical and psychological progress. Pain can interfere with sleep and eating, and further undermine the immune system (cancer already weakens immunity) leaving the patient open to infection. Constant pain rapidly changes a patient's attitude, causing anxiety, feelings of helplessness and hopelessness, and depression. In the worst case scenario, cancer pain can lead to suicide, and is a big factor driving the controversy over euthanasia. The good news is that most cancer pain is controllable by drug therapy. The mainstay is morphine, but even aspirin and paracetamol may play a role. The tragedy is that maybe half of all cancer patients suffer needless pain, because doctors and nurses too often misunderstand the nature of drugs such as morphine and underprescribe them. The way morphine works is discussed in more detail below.

Killing pain – how analgesics work

Painkilling drugs, such as aspirin and morphine, either stop the production of pain signals, or block their transmission to the brain. In medical jargon, they act either locally or centrally (the word central here refers to the central nervous system, comprising the brain and spinal cord).

Unlike most of the drugs discussed in this book, painkillers can be self-prescribed. Indeed, they are the best-selling category of over-the-counter medicines. The painkiller market in the UK alone is worth over £200 million a year (according to the latest figures), topping sales for both skin treatments and vitamins. Ninety per cent of people buy painkillers, and this percentage has been increasing over the years.

When surveyed by the manufacturers of the top-selling branded pain-killer, Nurofen (ibuprofen), people said the stresses and strains of modern life plus the effects of ageing accounted for increased consumption of pain-killers. What is more, most of us are going for the stronger, pharmacy only (P) painkillers, rather than those in the general sales list (GSL) category. Many painkillers are combinations of two drugs. For instance, Nurofen Plus, the strongest painkiller you can buy over the counter, is ibuprofen and codeine, while Solpadeine, Nurofen's nearest rival, is a combination of paracetamol, codeine and caffeine. Of all the ingredients of painkillers, paracetamol has had the main market share for several years, and now this stands at around 30 per cent.

Over-the-counter painkillers include both locally-acting and centrally-acting drugs. People use them for everyday aches and pains which they would not usually consult the doctor for — such as tension headache, period pains, backache, and the aches and pains of colds or flu. Incidentally, there is no real evidence that combination painkillers are more effective than single drugs.

The most commonly used locally-acting painkillers today are aspirin, paracetamol, and ibuprofen. And there are around 50 or so similar drugs. Even this is a bit of an oversimplification, because there is evidence that aspirin also has some central action, while no one is sure how paracetamol — the most popular single painkiller, remember — actually works at all.

The most important category of locally-acting painkillers is the non-steroidal anti-inflammatory agents, or NSAID. There are six different chemical classes of NSAID. Aspirin is a salicylate, while ibuprofen is in the class called propionic acid, and mefenamic acid, which is often prescribed for period pain and heavy menstrual bleeding, is a fenamate. Paracetamol is not an NSAID.

The NSAIDs attack the whole spectrum of pain, fever, and inflammation. Therefore they are used against colds and flu, as well as arthritis and related conditions. The key mode of action of the NSAIDs appears to be blocking of the production of prostaglandins, the hormones which mediate pain and inflammatory reactions — as has been discussed in previous chapters. How-ever, the amounts taken differ depending on whether the aim is to relieve pain or inflammation. For instance, the dose of aspirin needed to relieve pain is 1–3 grams a day while the dose to relieve the inflammation of, say, a swollen joint, is 4–8 grams a day. However, aspirin is not always the NSAID of choice in arthritis – and some patients with osteoarthritis manage perfectly well on paracetamol.

As has been mentioned in previous chapters, aspirin and other NSAIDs which block prostaglandin production, may cause serious side effects such as stomach bleeding and ulcers. Worse, the analgesic effects of the drugs may mask the symptoms of these problems – delaying treatment, an outcome which is potentially fatal. The reason for the side effects is that drugs that work by inhibition of prostaglandins lack specificity. Yes, prostaglandins act on nerve endings to produce pain, but other prostaglandins are responsible for the production of the protective mucus that lines the stomach. Further, asthmatics may be allergic to aspirin and it may, occasionally, lead to a serious disorder called Reye's syndrome which causes brain and kidney damage, in the under-twelves.

The development of more specific NSAIDs, which only inhibit the cyclo-oxygenase enzyme (COX2) involved in pain and inflammation (leaving the 'housekeeping' forms in the stomach and elsewhere alone) has already been discussed. But there are other approaches which may spare aspirin consumers from gastric side effects. Giving aspirin with lethicin, a component of stomach mucus, has been shown to offset some of the potential damage and help heal the stomach lining. Also, John Walker and his team at the University of Calgary in Canada have tried tacking a nitroxybutyl group onto the aspirin molecule. This breaks down to nitric oxide (NO), a potent vasodilator (and currently a hot topic in biology for all sorts of other reasons) which clears out an accumulation of white blood cells in the capillaries. If left unchecked, these cells appear to induce stomach ulceration. In animal tests, Walker's formulation protects against stomach ulceration. Human trials are underway and aspirin–NO should be on the market within five years.

Now to paracetamol. This is not, as stated above, an NSAID but it is still the world's most popular painkiller. However, it has come under scrutiny recently because of its danger in overdose. In normal dosage, paracetamol is one of the safest drugs known; it can even be recommended to pregnant women. In overdose, it causes 115 deaths a year in the UK, according to the latest figures. More deaths are caused by psychotropic drugs, such as anti-depressants (see Chapter 8), but the easy availability of paracetamol is a cause for concern. There are around 70,000 paracetamol overdoses in the UK (out of 30 million packs of tablets sold) each year. Despite some claims to the contrary, it is not easy to take an accidental fatal overdose of paracetamol. Taking fewer than 40 tablets is almost never fatal, according to the UK Home Office. The instructions on the packet stress that you should not take more than four grams or eight standard tablets a day. It would be hard to take more than five times this amount without realising it. However, there could be a danger in taking medicines containing paracetamol (such as hot lemon drinks) alongside paracetamol.

The problem is that if you do take too many, there will be no symptoms for 24 to 36 hours. During this time paracetamol, which is innocuous in its own right, will turn into a toxic breakdown product which poisons the liver. For those who go for an aspirin overdose, it is hard to ingest enough to do harm without being sick. And even if you do, alarming symptoms set in soon enough for help to be summoned by those who just took the overdose on impulse, and did not intend suicide.

But with paracetamol, by the time symptoms set in – such as jaundice and coma – it may be too late to reverse the damage. Ironically, the psychological crisis may be past for those who took an impulsive overdose. But the consequences of their action are yet to be worked out in the body.

Even so, there are two effective antidotes – methionine and acetylcysteine – which enhance the liver's ability to deal with the paracetamol toxin. Fewer than one per cent of people who take a paracetamol overdose die and even one in four of those in a coma recover with treatment. However, for some of those with liver failure, a transplant may be the only answer. Given the shortage of donor organs, it is hardly surprising that some clinicians and patient groups are calling for restriction on paracetamol sales to remove this particular source of demand.

There is a form of paracetamol, Pameton, which contains its own built-in antidote, cysteine. Although it is available over the counter, you cannot get it on the NHS because doctors have never accepted a clinical need for it. They argue that people who are determined on suicide will avoid Pameton and find some other drug to overdose with. Now the UK Medicines Control Agency has placed restrictions upon the sales of paracetamol. Supermarkets, garages and other general sales outlets will only be allowed to sell 12 tablets at a time. Pharmacies will be able to sell up to 50 tablets per customer, but larger amounts will be available on prescription only. In practice, such restrictions may not deter those bent on overdosing (they will just collect packets from several chemists).

There have been calls to ban paracetamol – chiefly from those who have lost a family member to overdose. The evidence suggests that in these cases, the victim – or the family member who found them – probably underestimated the number of tablets taken. It is unlikely that such a safe and effective drug would be taken off the market on the basis of such anecdotal evidence.

The centrally-acting opiates and opioids are the other main category of painkiller. Sometimes these are known as narcotics. This term has come to have criminal connotations (of which more in Chapter 9), but clinically it means drugs which depress the central nervous system, leading to stupor, loss of consciousness, and pain relief. Opiates are drugs derived from the opium poppy *Papaverum somniferum*. Opium itself has been used for pain relief for at least 2000 years, from the time of the ancient Romans. It was even mentioned in the Ebers papyrus, the first medical text, in 1550 BC, as a remedy for crying children, and there is evidence that it was known to the Sumerians as far back as 4000 BC, although we do not know what they used it for.

Opium is made from extracting the milky juice from the unripe seedpod of the poppy and letting it dry to a gum. Laudanum, a solution of opium in alcohol, became a popular all-purpose drug all over Europe by the 16th century, and trade in opium around the world was brisk.

Morphine is the major active ingredient of opium. It was isolated by the German pharmacist Friedrich Sertürner in the early 19th century. Typically, opium contains around 20 per cent morphine. In 1832, a second constituent of opium, codeine, was identified – but at levels around one tenth that of morphine. With the development of the hypodermic syringe, people began to inject morphine for both pain relief, and for its mood-altering qualities. Studies of the chemistry of morphine led to the synthesis of related drugs, known as the opioids. Diamorphine, commonly known as heroin, is the best-known of the opioids, which also include methadone and fentanyl. Heroin breaks down to morphine in the body and was in fact the first example of a pro-drug. Although it has strong analgesic properties it is unfortunately highly addictive.

In the field of strong pain relief, morphine remains the gold standard. It can be administered in many ways – orally, by injection, or by rectal suppository – which makes it very versatile. It brings powerful relief from both pain and anxiety. Therefore it is extremely valuable for treating the severe pain of heart attack, burns and cancer. It is also used for post-operative pain.

As with those other drug successes, aspirin and penicillin, the mode of action of morphine was not understood until many years after it first came into use. The opioids and opiates act as agonists on so-called μ-opioid receptors in the spinal cord and block the transmission of pain messages to the brain. There are also μ-opioid receptors in the brain, which may account for the mood-altering and addictive properties of the opiates and opioids. These receptors were only discovered in the 1970s. They are the sites of action of the body's natural painkillers, the endorphins (the name is short for endogenous morphine, or 'morphine produced from within'). One of these, β-endorphin, is 100 times stronger than morphine as a painkiller. Endorphin production within the brain after trauma may account for how soldiers often carry on fighting in battle despite severe injury, seemingly unaware of their pain. The release of endorphins is thought to account for the 'high' that sometimes accompanies jogging, meditation, and other 'feel good' activities. Endorphins may also play a role in the healing effect of acupuncture, or even in the placebo effect that often results from taking a dummy pill in a clinical trial. Two other classes of opioid receptor – the κ and δ receptors – have been discovered within the central nervous system. These are acted on by two other groups of naturally occurring substances – dynorphins and enkephalins, respectively. There is also some crossover between the activities of the three groups of agonists and their receptors, with dynorphins having some activity on μ-opioid receptors also, for example, while morphine appears to bind to a certain extent to all three types (although it is the interaction with the μ-opioid type which leads to pain relief).

The endorphins, enkephalins and dynorphins have quite different chemical structures from the opiates and opioids. They are peptides – short strings of amino acids – whereas morphine and its relations are alkaloids, smallish molecules which contain rings of nitrogen and carbon atoms. Recently two new endorphins, endomorphin-1 and endomorphin-2, which have great affinity and specificity for the μ-opioid receptor, have been discovered. But the endorphins are not used clinically because their lifetime in the body is too short.

Because opioid receptors have been found elsewhere in the body other than in the central nervous system, morphine has a number of side effects. It causes severe constipation, because of its effect on receptors affecting the ability of the gut to move its contents along, nausea and vomiting, dizziness, and contraction of the pupils of the eyes. However, these side effects do tend to decrease with time.

Even though morphine is the painkilling drug par excellence it is not as widely used as it might be. Many doctors and nurses appear to misunderstand morphine's effects. Mainly, they fear patients will become psychologically addicted to it (even if this were true, it would be hardly likely to cause any social problems in some of the patients who have most need of it – say, people with cancer who may have only weeks or days to live). However, the physical dependence which morphine induces is not the same as addiction. When someone is physically dependent on a drug, they suffer withdrawal symptoms when the drug is stopped. This is true of morphine in analgesia – withdrawal symptoms include diarrhoea and increased breathing rate. However, there is a psychological component to addiction which leads to craving and drug-seeking behaviour. When a patient no longer has a clinical need for morphine, it is very rare for this craving to develop. Another worry is that patients will become tolerant of the drug – requiring ever-increasing doses to obtain the same analgesic effect. Again, this is not addiction, although it is linked to physical dependence (all this is discussed in more detail in Chapter 9). Tolerance to morphine does occur, particularly to some of its side effects.

Patient surveys carried out by pain expert Ronald Melzack of McGill University in Montreal suggest that tolerance only actually occurs in around five per cent of patients treated with morphine. And a study of over 10,000 burns victims on morphine showed that not a single case of addiction could be attributed to its use (22 of the patients abused drugs after leaving hospital, but all had had a problem beforehand). Melzack and his team uncovered the reason for this in experiments on rats. They suggest that morphine acts on two different pain signalling pathways. One produces sharp, brief pain – like that of a cut finger – while the other produces the longer-lasting pain found in cancer. When morphine acts on this second pathway, it does not lead to great problems of tolerance or addiction.

If more doctors – and patients, who tend to share the fear of addiction – revised their view they might use morphine differently. Not just more often, but they might also adopt the dosing schedule developed by the English physician Cicely Saunders and other pioneers in palliative care (a term used mainly in cancer, referring to giving relief from pain and other symptoms, but without curing the disease). In this schedule morphine is given every four to six hours or on some other regular schedule, without waiting until the patient complains of pain. The revival of the Brompton cocktail – a mixture of gin, cocaine, morphine and chloroform, first used in the 19th century – has been another important development in palliative care.

The new Brompton cocktail is a liquid morphine beverage which relieves pain in 90 per cent of cancer patients (the dying British playwright Dennis Potter sipped it as he gave his lucid and coherent final TV interview in 1994). And half of those who still have pain can get relief if other ingredients are added to the cocktail. Patients can also use pumps, or slow-release capsules of morphine which give them much-desired control over their pain. These enlightened measures allow cancer and other terminal patients to spend their last weeks in dignity and comfort. Unfortunately, this relief is still not universally available. There is also evidence, from Melzack's studies, that painkillers are underprescribed in both children and the elderly and in burns patients. Morphine need not be kept only for cancer, burns and post-surgery – it can also be effective in the chronic 'useless' pain that persists for years after nerve injuries.

Sometimes the problem of pain can be addressed using drugs which are not, strictly speaking, analgesics. In recent years, it has been shown that both anti-depressant drugs and the anti-convulsants (normally used to treat epilepsy) can treat certain types of pain. The tricyclic anti-depressants (of which more in Chapter 8) such as amitryptiline are especially effective in treating pain occurring as a result of nerve damage. Tricyclics are also good for relieving chronic headache – especially the kind which is made worse by painkillers such as paracetamol. When anti-depressants are used to treat depression – at doses higher than those which are effective at killing pain – they do so by increasing levels of two brain chemicals, serotonin and noradrenaline. These are both neurotransmitters, and help neurons to communicate with one another. They are thought to be deficient in depression, and other types of mental illness, and anti-depressants restore levels and get the brain functioning normally again. But serotonin and noradrenaline are also involved in the transmission of pain signals. Although the painkilling properties of anti-depressants are not well understood, it is likely that they act by blocking pain signals in the spinal cord by acting on the serotonin and noradrenaline systems.

In trigeminal neuralgia, the branched nerve that runs up the face from the jaw to the eye is massively oversensitive to even the slightest stimulus. A gentle touch is felt like a knife in the face to someone with this condition, and they are likely to cry out with pain. It resembles epilepsy in the sense that there is excess electrical activity in the nerve fibres. In this sense, the shooting pain of trigeminal neuralgia and the convulsions of epilepsy have a common origin. So it is hardly surprising that the anti-convulsant drug carbamazepine is the treatment *par excellence* for trigeminal neuralgia.

But none of the painkillers discussed above is ideal, so pharmacologists are always on the look-out for new drugs. One which looks especially promising is epibatidine, which comes from glands on the back of the brightly coloured and poisonous Ecuador tree frog *Epibatides tricolor*. Animal tests suggest that epibatidine is 200 times stronger, as a painkiller, than morphine. It looks as if the drug may act in a different way from the opiates – although the exact mechanism is not yet fully understood.

Only a few milligrams of epibatidine are obtainable from several hundred frogs. So for both practical and conservation reasons, a lab synthesis is necessary if the drug is to make any headway. But the epibatidine molecule itself is unusual for one that occurs in nature – it contains a chlorine atom, and a six-membered carbon ring bridged by a nitrogen atom. This makes its synthesis a bit of a challenge, but it has now been done by Mark Trudell and Chunming Zhang of the University of New Orleans. They are confident that their method lends itself to scale-up – a limitation of previous attempts to synthesise epibatidine.

Out and under – the science of anaesthesia

Until the discovery of anaesthetics in the 19th century, surgery was a brutal and risky affair which would only be undertaken if absolutely necessary. Then an American doctor, William Thomas Morton, began experimenting with ether, showing that it induced unconsciousness. He used it to extract a tooth on September 30 1846 and then, on October 16 in the same year removed a tumour from a patient under ether. The next year chloroform was introduced. But both of these early anaesthetics had their hazards. Chloroform is toxic to the liver, while ether is highly flammable.

However, one of the original anaesthetics, nitrous oxide, is still in use today. The gas was discovered by Joseph Priestley in 1772, and was soon known for its intoxicant effects which earned it the name laughing gas. Soon people were indulging in laughing gas 'parties' and roadshow demonstrations. A young American dentist, Horace Wells, noticed how a volunteer at one of these demonstrations fell heavily into a table without flinching and saw immediately how to exploit the pain-numbing effects of the gas. He pioneered its use in dentistry, and it is the mainstay of general surgical anaesthesia to this day.

General anaesthesia is reversible drug-induced loss of awareness and sensation characterised by a general depression of neuronal activity. In itself, this causes unwanted physiological effects like excessive salivation and a decrease in the heart rate. These are countered by giving a so-called muscarinic antagonist, such as atropine, along with a tranquilliser such as valium to decrease anxiety. Then a quick-acting intravenous drug such as thiopentone sodium, a barbiturate, is given. The main anaesthetic is usually inhaled as a mixture of, say, 50 to 70 per cent nitrous oxide with one per cent of halothane, a volatile liquid. Enflurane or isoflurane are newer anaesthetics which might be used in place of halothane.

It may sound scary, but no one is really sure how general anaesthetics work. It probably has something to do with the way the anaesthetic molecules interact with the fatty membranes of neurones, which appears to decrease transmission of messages between the cells. In fact, any organic solvent would probably act as an anaesthetic for this reason – but most are far too toxic.

Local anaesthetics such as lidocaine, which are used to numb the mouth during dental surgery, for instance, are better understood. These seem to block the primary pain signals and make minor surgery, dentistry, and even injections less traumatic.

The problem of pain, therefore, can be addressed by a wide spectrum of drugs. Most often the solution – aspirin or paracetamol – is cheap, readily available, and highly effective. And for those with severe pain, there is always the comfort offered by morphine – if doctor and patient can overcome any groundless fears about its use. In this chapter we have touched upon the pain of cancer; in the next we survey the difficult issue of how to treat cancer with drugs.

7

The cancer challenge

Cancer is probably the biggest current challenge to the pharmaceutical industry. One person in three will be diagnosed with cancer during their lifetime in the Western world and fewer than half can expect a complete cure. This is despite the hundreds of millions of dollars spent on research and treatments over the last 30 years or so.

And cancer is an increasing problem; the World Health Organization predicts a 40 per cent increase in cancer cases over the next 25 years in the West, and a doubling in developing countries. According to a recent report commissioned by the charity Macmillan Cancer Relief, one Briton in two can expect to contract cancer in their lifetime by 2018 (compared to one in three today).

There are also marked trends in certain types of cancer. Currently lung cancer is the commonest fatal cancer in men. It could be overtaken by prostate cancer by the next century, however. Male lung cancer rates are falling, while prostate cancer has doubled over the last 20 years. On the other hand, female lung cancer is increasing. It could soon overtake breast cancer as the leading cause of cancer death in women. Malignant melanoma, a skin cancer, is on the increase in both men and women, while stomach cancer continues to decrease.

Doctors have a good idea what lies behind at least some of these trends; food preservatives (despite their bad press in some quarters) are generally accepted to protect us from toxins in food that could otherwise trigger a stomach cancer. Changes in the incidence of lung cancer can largely be accounted for by changes in smoking behaviour in men and women. And increased exposure to the sun from a combination of cheap package holidays in hot countries and a decrease in protection from sunlight from the thinning ozone layer makes a major contribution to the greater incidence of melanoma. The majority of cancers are probably preventable (Table 2). But it is hard to persuade people to change their behaviour and where diet, for instance, is concerned, it is not really yet known what advice people should be given.

Looking at the cancer statistics may lead you to believe that medical research has a very poor record at providing drug therapies that can cure. That conclusion might be a little unfair. Some cancers, such as testicular cancer and childhood leukaemias, are now almost 100 per cent curable with anti-cancer drugs. British cancer expert John Cairns, now professor of public health at Harvard, reckons that between 5 and 10 per cent of cancers that would have been fatal 20 years ago are now cured by drug therapy. Even so, many patients claim that treatment with anti-cancer drugs is worse than the symptoms of the disease itself. So the pharmaceutical industry still has much to do.

However, the future looks bright. Advances in molecular biology technique are revolutionising our understanding of how cancer arises in the body. These new insights have led to the development of hundreds of potential new drugs which promise a clean break with the blunderbuss approach of today's cancer therapies.

Cancer starts in the genes

In the mid-1950s Howard Temin, of Caltech in Pasadena, carried out a groundbreaking experiment in cancer research. It has long been known that certain viruses are able to cause tumours in animals (including humans, as was later discovered), but the mechanism remained obscure. Temin mixed cancer virus particles with chicken cells in a Petri dish and showed that the viruses made the cells multiply out of control – a process known as transformation. Temin's experiment showed that cancer occurs at the level of the cell, rather than the tissue or organ. It also focused attention on the fact that viruses do not cause cancer by killing cells. Instead they, and other cancer inducing agents, cause tumours by transforming normal cells into cancer cells.

Normal cells behave completely differently from cancer cells. They act as law-abiding members of a community, responding to signals from their neighbours and their general environment which tell them when to multiply and when to stay quiescent. They have a finite life, measured out by the number of times they can divide. And if they become badly damaged, they normally do the decent thing and kill themselves in a process known as apoptosis.

Cancer cells, in contrast, ignore these checks and balances. They multiply continually, forming tumour masses. They seem able to evade the discipline of apoptosis and can break away from the site of the tumour and colonise the rest of the body.

Over the last 20 years or so, the main thrust of cancer research has been to understand how cancer cells can behave in this antisocial and undisciplined way. It is now evident that mutations in genes that control cell division drive the cancer process. This kind of understanding would not have been possible before the development of technologies to study DNA and genes in the 1970s and 1980s. To date 20 or so genes involved in cancer have been discovered. Homing in on the disease at a molecular level in this way is excellent news – for it opens up the possibility of cleaner and more effective anti-cancer drugs.

There are two main classes of cancer genes which are being worked on – proto-oncogenes, and tumour suppressor genes. The proto-oncogenes stimulate cell division while tumour suppressors, as the name suggests, inhibit it. Should any of these genes become mutated, the fine control of cell division control may be disrupted. Cancer is not inevitable at this stage – as will be discussed below – as the cell is likely to repair the damage.

The best-understood of the proto-oncogenes is called *ras*, which has been the subject of intense study for around 15 years. The protein encoded by a normal *ras* gene stands at the head of a chain of command starting outside a cell, and ending at its control centre, the nucleus (Fig. 7.1). The ras molecule can bind to the small molecules GTP and GDP, and in so doing it acts as a kind of molecular switch with the GTP-bound state corresponding to 'on' and the GDP-bound state corresponding to 'off'. In the 'on' state, it can relay signals down the chain to the nucleus, but in the 'off' state the signal is not transmitted. Typically, this signal comes from a hormone known as a growth factor, when it docks onto a receptor on the cell surface (see also Chapter 4 for more about how hormones control the activities of cells). The act of docking turns ras 'on' and the signal to divide is relayed to the nucleus, which activates genes involved in the cell division process. If division is inappropriate, the growth factor receptor is unoccupied and the relay system falls silent, allowing the cell to rest.

But if *ras* is mutated, the protein is frozen in the 'on' position and the relay system hums continuously, forcing the cell to divide over and over again in the absence of any external growth factor signals. This is cancer in the making. Mutated *ras* genes (known as oncogenes, whereas the normal versions are called proto-oncogenes) are found in one-third of all human

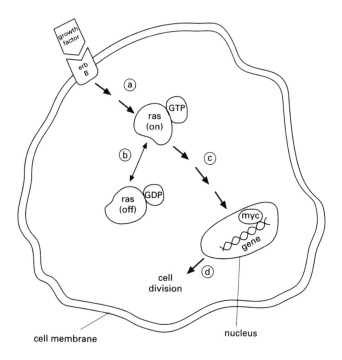

Fig. 7.1. How gene mutations can cause cancer. In an idealised cancer cell (not all the genes and proteins discussed here will be active in all cancer cells) a growth factor docks onto a membrane-bound receptor, erb-B. This triggers a chain of biochemical signals (a) which switch ras protein into its 'on' position. When erb-B is mutated this chain is activated whether or not growth factor is present. Ras switches between the 'on' and 'off' positions (b) depending on whether it receives a signal from the receptor. But if ras is mutated it becomes jammed into the 'on' position. When in the 'on' position, a message is relayed to the nucleus (c) which causes proteins such as myc to activate genes involved in cell division (d). Mutated versions of myc switch these genes on inappropriately.

cancers, and are especially common in carcinomas of the colon, lung and pancreas (indeed they have been found in nearly every pancreatic tumour studied to date). Carcinomas are the most common form of cancer, and originate in the epithelial cells, which line body cavities.

Evidence is emerging that other proteins in the relay system are mutated in cancer, from the growth factor receptors to the proteins at the end of the line, the transcription factors which turn on the genes in the nucleus. For instance, the gene *erb-B* which encodes the receptor for epidermal growth factor (one of the important growth factors), is often mutated in breast cancer and in glioblastoma, a form of brain cancer. Watch out too for news of a gene called *myc*, whose encoded protein turns on cell-division genes. Mutated *myc* genes have been detected in breast, lung, stomach and nerve cell cancers, as well as in some leukaemias and glioblastoma.

Also important are mutations in *bcl*, a gene which codes for a protein which helps cells evade apoptosis. Under normal conditions, *bcl* does a vital job; like cell division, apoptosis must be kept in balance – if it happens when it should not, cells kill themselves off uncessarily (it seems that excessive apoptosis may be responsible for tissue damage that follows heart attack or stroke). Cancer cells, being abnormal, are obvious candidates for apoptosis. However, levels of *bcl* in cancer cells are often higher than normal, suggesting that the cells are able to evade apoptosis.

Rampant cell division is normally brought under control by one or more of the proteins coded for by the tumour suppressor genes. These work in a similar way to the relay system described above, only they convey inhibitory, rather than activating, signals. One of the key tumour suppressor genes is called *p*53. It halts cell division, and causes damaged cells (such as cancer cells) to undergo apoptosis. Half of all human tumours studied lack a functional *p*53 protein, because the corresponding gene is mutated.

Robert Weinberg of the Massachusetts Institute of Technology has developed a new picture of how cancer happens, based upon what we now know of the role genes play (Fig. 7.2) (Weinberg himself was involved in the isolation of both the first human oncogene and the first human tumour suppressor gene.) The main feature of this model is that a tumour results from the accumulation of, say, half a dozen or so different mutations in a tissue and typically, takes many years to develop (cancer is, by and large, a disease of older people).

First, a mutation of the type described above occurs in a single cell within a tissue. What causes this mutation? A mutation is a 'mistake' within the DNA sequence of a gene. There are several different kinds of mutation and here we will just discuss a so-called point mutation, in which just a single letter in the DNA code is 'wrong' (like mistyping 'hare' instead of 'here'). Point mutations occur in a number of ways. From time to time they arise spontaneously in the cell, when it has to copy its genes just before cell division. Just like copy typing, mistakes will be made. Or some external agent, such as a virus or chemical, may home in on the DNA and cause a mutation (for most of the causes of cancer listed in Table 2 a mechanism of damaging DNA in this way has been worked out). Occasionally people are

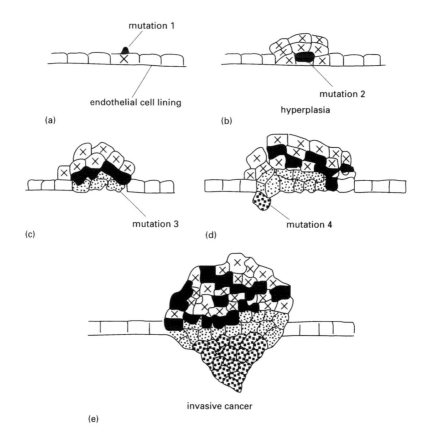

Fig. 7.2. The route to cancer. An endothelial cell is mutated (a) in such a way
as to let it divide more rapidly than normal cells. This leads to an overgrowth
of these cells (b) known as hyperplasia. Sooner or later one of these cells takes
a second mutation hit. Again, these cells multiply at an abnormally high rate,
giving rise to a more obvious state of overgrowth called dysplasia (c). A third
mutation leads, again through abnormal cell division, to a tumour located at
the site of the original mutation (d) known as *in situ* cancer. A fourth mutation
(e) may allow the tumour to invade neighbouring tissue and, eventually, to
metastasise throughout the body.

born with a mutation in a cancer gene. Mostly all these mutations are
repaired by enzymes within the cell. If they are not, then the affected cell
differs from its neighbours in having a tendency to divide where they would
rest.

Over a period of time, a population of these cells develops and after a

Table 2. *The causes of cancer*[a]

Cause	Percentage of all cancer cases[b]
Familial (i.e. inheritance of a cancer gene)	5
Arising naturally within the body (no external carcinogen or inherited gene involved)	25
Smoking	30
Diet (high consumption of red meat and animal fats, low consumption of fruit and vegetables, obesity)	30
Alcohol	3
Sedentary lifestyle	3
Food additives (mainly salt)	1
Viral infection	5
Radiation (mainly sunlight and radon)	2
Workplace chemicals	5
Environmental pollutants	2
Medical treatments (e.g. immune suppressant and hormonal drugs)	1

[a]Data refers to the US and other industrial nations
[b]Figures add to more than 100 because of rounding and overlapping of causes

while, one of them acquires a second mutation which further loosens the controls over cell division. Next, a third mutation is acquired and this population expands even more. By this stage, some abnormalities may become apparent in the mutated cells when they are examined under the microscope; these are the types of changes which are sometimes picked up in cells by a cervical smear test. Clinically, this is called carcinoma *in situ*. This tiny tumour may not progress for years – or at all. The person affected may die of some other cause and never be aware that he or she has had cancer.

However, if the *in situ* tumour goes on to acquire one or more mutations which give it additional growth advantage the tumour may start to invade surrounding tissue. At this stage the tumour would be classified as malignant. It may also shed cells into the bloodstream which can establish new tumours elsewhere in the body – a process known as metastasis.

People who inherit mutations in cancer genes start off with an obvious disadvantage. They are more likely to acquire those second and third mutations than people who start off with normal versions of the genes, and so progress to a cancer at a younger age (and, of course, their risk of getting cancer at all is dramatically increased). For instance, inheritance of a mutated form of a tumour suppressor gene called APC leads to a condition called familial adenomatous polyposis (FAP), characterised by multiple polyps in the colon. Over time, these polyps become cancerous. And the two breast cancer genes which have hit the headlines recently, BRCA1 and BRCA2, are likely also be be tumour supressor genes.

How cancer spreads

Cancers that stay *in situ* are are far easier to deal with clinically than those which have begun to roam the body. Therefore, better understanding of the mechanisms of metastasis is a great step forward and is already leading to new treatments which enable a patient to 'live with' a cancer, by limiting its spread, rather than eradicating it from the body.

Just as there are controls over cell division, so there are also checks on keeping cells in their place within a tissue. Malignant cancer cells have found ways of evading these checks. Normal cells stick to one another in a tissue, and also to the extracellular matrix – the biological 'glue' which moulds individual cells into a block of tissue. Recent discoveries have shown that cell adhesion molecules (CAMs), which occur on the cell surface, are largely responsible for making sure that a cell is in the right place, and that it stays there. In cancer cells, CAMs are either absent, or altered. For instance, blocking a key CAM called E–cadherin makes normal cells invasive in test-tube experiments; the reverse occurs if it is added to cells which lack it – they switch from being invasive to non-invasive.

Another important group of CAMs are the integrins, which anchor cells to the extracellular matrix. If a cell does not anchor, it undergoes apoptosis. Cancer cells appear to be anchorage-independent, so if they trespass on new tissue by metastasis they establish themselves. It is thought that this may happen by oncogenes sending out false signals to the apoptosis apparatus, pretending that the cells are anchored when they are not.

The picture which is emerging of metastasis is as follows: a cancer cell leaves its tissue of origin and burrows through its basement membrane (the structure which forms a boundary to the tissue). The only other cells which can escape in this way are white blood cells, which do so when summoned to a site of injury or infection by the immune system, of which they are a key part. Cancer cells have high levels of enzymes called matrix metalloprot-einases (MMPs) which can remodel the extracellular matrix by breaking down some of its component molecules such as collagen. The MMPs tunnel through the basement membrane and, once free, the cancer cell soon finds a blood vessel (any tissue not near a blood vessel would soon die for lack of oxygen and nutrients). Having worked its way through the basement membrane of the blood vessel, the cancer cell is now free to wander around the body, to find a new home in which to establish itself. Generally, it will get trapped in the first available vascular bed and find its way into nearby tissue. For most organs, this first port of call would be the lungs, except for the digestive organs, where it would be the liver. This explains why so many secondary tumours are found in lungs and liver.

Many of the details of the above journey of a cancer, from a mutation in a single cell to life-threatening stranglehold, remain to be worked out. But even the broad sweep offers ample targets for drug therapy. It is on this basis that the 21st century battle against cancer will be fought; existing therapy, as we will see, has developed largely without the knowledge outlined above.

Killing cancer – chemotherapy today

The idea that drugs might cure cancer came from observation of the effects of mustard gas on soldiers in World War I. Mustard gas, a form of chemical warfare, belongs to a group of compounds known as the alkylating agents which can severely damage DNA. No one knew about DNA in World War I, of course, but they did notice that men who died from mustard gas exposure had severely lowered levels of white blood cells. The rationale for trying chemical warfare agents as cancer chemotherapy was that white blood cell count rockets in some forms of cancer, such as leukaemia. Indeed, a nitrogen mustard, mustine, is still the mainstay – and a fairly successful one – of treatment for Hodgkin's disease, a cancer of the lymphatic system. But cancer chemotherapy did not really come into the mainstream of medicine until around the 1940s.

A few cancers, such as testicular cancer and some forms of leukaemia, are curable by drugs alone. However, for the more common cancers such as breast, lung, colo-rectal (large bowel or large intestine) and prostate, chemotherapy is only useful as part of a treatment programme. Surgery and radiotherapy can only treat *in situ* tumours. If the primary tumour is removed by one or both of these, then chemotherapy can follow to mop up any rogue cancer cells in the system which have metastasised. This follow-up chemotherapy has already been shown to improve the cure rate in both breast and colo-rectal cancer.

In some cancers, such as head and neck, lung, and bladder, the chemotherapy might come first to shrink a tumour before it is surgically removed or treated by radiotherapy. And sometimes chemotherapy is given alongside surgery or radiotherapy to get a better response in cancer of the oesophagus, which is hard to treat by surgery alone.

Most anti-cancer drugs act by damaging some component of the cancer cell so that it undergoes apoptosis and dies. Indeed, cancer cells with high levels of bcl protein, or which lack $p53$, are often resistant to chemotherapy – because they do not undergo apoptosis as readily as normal cells.

One of the most widely used drugs, methotrexate, blocks the enzyme dihydrofolate reductase (DHFR) which is needed to provide two of the vital building blocks of DNA, adenine and guanine. (An antibiotic, trimethoprim, which acts in the same way, was described in Chapter 3.) Without adenine and guanine DNA synthesis grinds to a halt.

The alkylating agents, such as mustine and cyclophosphamide, add methyl groups (a cluster of one carbon and three hydrogen atoms) at points along the cancer cell's DNA; this leads to chemical bonds breaking within the molecule, which in turn triggers apoptosis.

Another routinely used drug, doxorubicin, acts by getting between the building blocks of the DNA in a cancer cell, thereby stopping it producing the proteins it codes for. Such damage is almost certain to lead to the death of the cell by apoptosis. The antibiotic actinomycin, which is mainly used for childhood cancers these days, acts in a similar way (and was also discussed in Chapter 3).

A newer drug, cisplatin – which as the name suggests contains the precious metal platinum – also binds to DNA. It is useful mainly in testicular and ovarian cancer. Recent experiments have shown that a protein called hMSH2, which normally patrols DNA looking for problems to repair, sticks fast to cisplatin when it detects it on the molecule. However, the protein is unable to repair the strand once cisplatin is in place and the damaged cell is marked down for apoptosis. The hMSH2 protein occurs at high levels in the testes and ovary, which may explain why cisplatin is so effective in cancers of these organs; it may also point to ways of making cisplatin effective in other cancers, if ways to increase levels of hMSH2 in other tumours could be found.

Some anti-cancer drugs are natural products. Vincristine and vinblastine, which come from the Madagascan rosy periwinkle and are effective in curing childhood leukaemias, act on the cell's skeleton. This is made from a protein called tubulin which polymerises to form a network of microtubules. When the cell is resting these provide it with a supporting framework. And when it divides, they form a structure called the spindle which separates out the pairs of chromosomes (containing the genes) for delivery into the two new cells. Vincristine and vinblastine interfere with the formation of the cyto-skeleton by binding to tubulin.

One of the latest, and best-publicised, anti-cancer compounds is taxol (also known as paclitaxel) which is derived from the yew tree. Taxol also acts on tubulin, but by 'freezing' the cytoskeleton so that the spindle cannot move the chromosomes into their new locations on cell division.

The original version of taxol came from the bark of the Pacific yew, an endangered species. It took the bark of two trees to provide enough taxol to treat one patient. A complete synthesis of taxol was worked out in 1994 by K. C. Nicolaou of the University of California. Unfortunately, this is not a practical option as it involves 30 stages with a yield of less than five per cent from its starting material. Nowadays taxol is made by a semi-synthetic process; the needles (a renewable resource) of the Western yew provide an intermediate which can be transformed to taxol in the laboratory. There is also a synthetic analogue of taxol called taxotere. Taxol is, so far, licensed for the treatment of breast, lung, ovarian and prostate cancer, as well as malignant melanoma and Kaposi's sarcoma (the skin cancer that often accompanies AIDS). Taxotere is used in breast and lung cancer. In one recent trial, 56 per of cent women with advanced breast cancer – for whom all other treatments had failed – gained an extra year of life on taxotere. Not a cure, of course, but probably of great value to the women and their families. Despite some side effects, many of these patients said they felt much better on the drug.

Cancers of the reproductive system, such as breast and prostate, grow under the influence of sex hormones (see also Chapter 4 for how hormones stimulate growth of tissue). These can be treated with compounds that block the action of these hormones. Tamoxifen, for example, blocks the action of oestrogen and is used both as treatment in breast cancer and, in an ongoing trial, as a preventative drug for women at high risk of developing the disease.

The two main problems with current cancer chemotherapy are the side effects and drug resistance. Side effects, which can be so severe that they lead to a patient refusing chemotherapy, arise from the fact that normal cells, as well as cancer cells, are affected by anti-cancer drugs. True, cancer cells *are* very different from normal cells. The problem is that where cytotoxic (cell-killing) drugs are concerned, they are not different enough. Rapidly dividing cells in the body, such as hair follicle cells, stem cells in bone marrow which give rise to blood cells, and the cells that line the digestive system are all hit nearly as hard by cytotoxic drugs as are the cancer cells themselves. The result is hair loss, lowered resistance to infection, anaemia, nausea and vomiting.

To an extent these side effects can be countered. Cooling the scalp during chemotherapy reduces the risk of hair loss. There are new drugs which can protect against side effects. For instance, a compound called stem cell protector is in phase II trials; it stops the stem cells dividing during chemotherapy so that they are not so much affected by the anti-cancer drug. And there are several drugs which alleviate nausea and vomiting by acting on the appropriate receptors in the brain's vomiting centre.

Ultimately, however, the best way of dealing with side effects might be to target the drug more effectively to cancer cells, leaving normal cells alone. This would allow doctors to increase the dosage of effective cytotoxic drugs in the hope of hitting a tumour harder.

One way of doing this is to fix the drug to a vehicle, such as a polymer, which also has a targetting group attached to it. The targetting group will home in on a molecule which is found on the surface of cancer cells, but not on normal cells, and so guide the drug to its target. What is more, such systems exploit the fact that the blood supply to tumours is more 'leaky' than that to normal cells. So more drug will get in compared to normal tissue. And cancer cells have no lymphatic drainage, so the drug cannot easily get out of the tissue. This so-called enhanced permeability retention (EPR) was discovered by Hiroshi Maeda, a Japanese researcher, in 1989. Trials of delivery of doxorubicin by this system show that 70 times more of the polymer-attached drug than the free drug can be delivered to a mouse melanoma. More significantly, human volunteers can tolerate a five times higher concentration of doxorubicin using this system than when it is administered by conventional means.

In place of polymers fixed with a targetting group, chemotherapy can be administered instead using a monoclonal antibody which will carry the drug to cancer cells. The toxic drug calicheamicin, a natural product, is enjoying a new lease of life, thanks to this technology. It is now in early clinical trials for leukaemia and ovarian cancer. Ricin, one of the most toxic molecules known, is also being hitched to antibodies for use as an anti-cancer drug. Other drugs being tested with this technology are maytansine, which is derived from an African plant, and a taxol derivative manufactured by American biotechnology giant Genentech.

Finally, there is Antibody Directed Enzyme Pro-drug Therapy (ADEPT) in which a monoclonal antibody takes an enzyme to the cancer cell where it converts a previously adminstered pro-drug into its active form. Normal cells are unaffected, as the antibody is directed only to the cancer cells.

As with antibiotic resistance (see also Chapter 3), drug resistance is a major problem in cancer chemotherapy. To an extent, this has been overcome by using a combination of drugs, on the same principle that drug 'cocktails' are used to combat infectious diseases such as AIDS (see Chapter 3). Many drug-resistant cancers have high levels of a molecule called p-glycoprotein, which pumps the drug out of cells. These 'guards' can be overcome by using drugs like verapamil, and more advanced analogues, which will smuggle the anti-cancer drug in through channels in the cell membrane.

New ways of combating cancer

The face of cancer chemotherapy could be transformed within the next 20 years, if even a fraction of the new drugs in the pipeline live up to their initial promise. Many are quite different from current cytotoxic drugs. Some stop a tumour from spreading, some mobilise or mimic the body's own defences against cancer, while others home in on cancer genes.

Probably the most advanced of these new drugs are the matrix metalloproteinase inhibitors (MMPIs). The matrix metalloproteinases (MMPs) are enzymes which are found at higher than normal levels in cancer cells. They are deeply implicated in the growth and spread of tumours, for they etch a path for cancer cells through the surrounding tissue by digesting the collagen molecules that hold the tissue together. If this action can be checked by an inhibitor molecule, then the cancer may become non-invasive and therefore less of a threat.

The MMP molecules contain zinc within their active site. The inhibitors are small molecules which bind to zinc and so stop the approach of the collagen substrate; an advantage is that they can be administered orally, so the patient can take them at home. The MMPIs have been studied since the early 1980s and there are now seven compounds in clinical trials. One of these, Marimastat – which has been developed by British Biotech – hit the headlines when it successfully came through phase II trials for ovarian, colo-rectal, prostate, gastric and pancreatic cancers. Treatment decreased levels of cancer antigens in the blood, used as a marker of the disease – so a reponse was seen at the biochemical level. It also increased survival of the patients to an extent which was shown to be statistically significant; however, remember, these patients – as in many cancer trials – had advanced disease and short life expectancy. It will take much more investigation to discover just how helpful Marimastat can be for the average cancer patient. Much – clinically and financially – hangs on the phase III results. British Biotech has launched the biggest ever drug trial for advanced pancreatic cancer involving 700 patients in the UK and the US, where Marimastat is being tested against the best existing treatment, a drug called gemcitabine.

Another way of stopping the spread of a tumour is to 'strangle' it by cutting off its blood supply. As a tumour grows, it needs to develop blood vessels to bring the cells within it nutrients and oxygen. The cells have been shown to secrete a substance called vascular endothelial growth factor (VEGF), which triggers angiogenesis – the growth of new blood vessels. Companies such as the US biotech major Genentech have shown that molecules that target both VEGF itself and its receptor on endothelial cells (which line existing blood vessels and provide a 'base' for the new blood supply) can slow or even halt the growth of tumours in mice. Better still, adult humans do not need VEGF as their normal blood supply is fully developed. So these new drugs should leave normal tissue alone.

Judah Folkman at Harvard Medical School, who has been at the forefront of research into angiogenesis, has recently announced the discovery of endostatin, a molecule which occurs naturally in cells. Endostatin, and related compounds such as thrombospondin and angiostatin, have the ability to inhibit angiogenesis. What is particularly interesting is that thrombospondin appears to be controlled by the tumour suppressor p53 – so maybe this natural 'strangulation' process is one way in which the body uses its defences to keep cancers from taking hold. And in a suprising comeback, thalidomide has been shown to have anti-cancer properties by inhibiting angiogenesis in mice. The exact mechanism is unknown. But since angiogenesis is needed for the normal development of limbs in the embryo, this discovery may shed light on why thalidomide had such disastrous effects on unborn children when it was in general use (see Chapter 1).

And there is a third approach; you can stop blood flowing to tumours in its existing blood supply. A natural blood clotting molecule called tissue factor linked to a tumour-targetting molecule can cause tiny blood clots to form just in the vessels supplying the tumour. Finally, there is much excitement over another potential drug of this kind – combretastatin, which has been extracted from the bark of the South African bush willow *Combretum caffrum*. While the exact mechanism of combretastatin's action remains unclear, it certainly cuts off the blood supply to breast tumours in mice within 20 minutes. Within 24 hours, 95 per cent of the tumour cells were dead – showing the potency of this approach to cancer therapy. The research into combretastatin has been backed by the UK Cancer Research Campaign, and it is hoped that the drug will be applicable to all types of cancer.

There has been much interest in new drugs that stimulate apoptosis in cancer cells. Two surprising candidates in this category are aspirin and a traditional Chinese remedy containing arsenic trioxide. It has long been known that regular consumption of aspirin for relief of other conditions, such as arthritis, halves the incidence of bowel cancer. Sulindac, another NSAID, decreases the incidence of bowel polyps in familes with FAP (a condition which, as described earlier, usually progresses to cancer). Now a study of bowel cancer cells and aspirin and sulindac has shown that the drugs slow the growth of the cells, and also make some of them undergo apoptosis. Before long, doctors could be recommending aspirin as a preventative against bowel cancer – at least in those at most risk – and maybe for oesophageal and gastric cancer too. For some unknown reason, aspirin and related compounds only appear to be effective against cancers of the digestive tract.

The development of arsenic trioxide as an anti-cancer drug started when doctors in north-east China were ordered by Mao Tse-Tung to prove the superiority of Chinese traditional medicine over Western practices. The arsenic-containing remedy, which had been in use for thousands of years against arthritis and skin disorders, was found to be surprisingly effective in terminal leukaemia, producing long-lasting remissions. Recent laboratory experiments showed that arsenic trioxide induces apoptosis in cancer cells. Now researchers in Shanghai plan to test the drug in other tumours, and will also search through other Chinese traditional remedies for more compounds that can induce apoptosis.

The idea of vaccinating against cancer may seem far-fetched; we normally associate vaccination with infectious disease. In fact it has long been known that the immune system will attack cancer cells (after all, like invading bacteria and viruses, they are 'foreign'). Paul Ehrlich carried out many experiments in which he created infections in animals with tumours. Often this would clear the cancer, presumably by rousing the animal's immune system. Further, people on long-term immunosuppressant drugs such as cyclosporin (to stop transplanted organs such as kidneys and hearts being rejected) appear to have a higher rate of cancer than the rest of the population. But the immune system is not completely successful in attacking cancer cells, because they themselves often secrete immunosuppressants (such as a molecule called transforming growth factor (TGF) β) which will thwart any such attack.

These days, the vaccination approach depends upon discovering the molecules on the surface of cancer cells which make them look 'foreign'. An effective vaccine would be targetted against these molecules, which are known as tumour-associated antigens. Several of these antigens have already been discovered, by extracting tumour cells from patients and analysing them.

A cancer vaccine involves injecting these antigen molecules into the patient. The immune system recognises them as 'foreign' and so mounts an attack, producing neutralising antibodies, and rousing T cells which will chew up any cell which displays the antigen. Once primed like this, the immune system should turn its attention to the antigen-labelled tumour cell. Of course, the immune system may have mounted its own attack on the cancer, without the vaccine. But if the tumour is growing, this attack has not been enough. Administering the vaccine will enhance the immune response to the tumour. Experimental vaccines are now in phase II trials for end stage breast, colon, and pancreatic cancers. In colo-rectal cancer, there has been a small, but significant increase in five year survival from 27 per cent to 30 per cent.

It is now clear that some cancers are caused by viruses. These are the obvious target for vaccination and several companies are developing vaccines against papilloma virus, for instance.

Some of the newer anti-cancer drugs, such as interferon and interleukin-2, are molecules which are naturally produced by the body. They are, broadly speaking, components of the immune system which can be useful, like vaccines, in boosting the defences against cancer. These are produced by genetic engineering (and so will be discussed further in Chapter 11).

The prospects for the future of cancer chemotherapy look very bright. New drugs will be based on the deeper understanding of the disease which has come from the research efforts of the last 20 years. But as with cardiovascular disease, drugs alone will not beat cancer. People can make lifestyle changes, such as stopping smoking or eating a better diet, which may ensure that they never have need of anti-cancer therapies.

So far we have reviewed drugs which act on physical disease. But much ill health comes from mental illness. In the next chapter we look at drugs which aim to heal mental disorder by acting on the brain.

8

Drugs for the mind

No one denies the reality of infection, heart disease, pain or cancer – or questions the scientific rationale behind the design of drugs to relieve or cure these conditions. With mental illnesses, such as depression and schizophrenia, the situation is a little different. The development and use of pharmaceutical drugs which work on the mind is one of the most controversial areas in medicine today (recreational drugs work on the mind too, and are also the subject of controversy. We will look at these in the next chapter).

If you flip through the pages of the Diagnostic and Statistical Manual IV (commonly known as DSM IV) you might think that psychiatry is as cut and dried a scientific discipline as any other branch of clinical medicine. DSM IV is the American Association of Psychiatry's classification of mental illness and on first glance it looks as authoritative and impressive as the Oxford Textbook of Medicine. A closer look reveals some curious – and fascinating – mental diseases. What about 'oppositional defiant disorder' and 'bereavement reaction'? Here the normal spectrum of human behaviour (childhood disobedience and grief, respectively) appear to undergo a subtle shift into psychological pathology. Classification of physical disease is usually more clear-cut.

For most of the mental conditions in DSM IV there is no physical diagnosis such as a blood test or scan, which also sets them aside from most physical diseases. An exception is Alzheimer's disease, which – as we shall see – is associated with specific brain lesions, currently only detectable *post mortem*. Instead of running lab tests, psychiatrists and family doctors rely on their own observations and questioning the patient. Even so, drugs are frequently used in treating mental illnesses and are often remarkably effective – in depression, for instance, or at least make the patient's condition (cynics would say the patient) more manageable, as in schizophrenia.

Such drugs, which affect mind and mood, are known as psychotropics. They include tranquillisers, anti-depressants, and stimulants. They all act on the brain. The problem is that the brain is the least understood part of the body, and the relationship between brain and mind is complex and controversial. Although anti-depressants do lift mood (in about 70 per cent of cases, anyway), and we know quite a bit about how they affect the brain, there is no hard evidence that they really get to the root of the problem in the way an antibiotic clears an infection. Or to put it in the words of psychologist Dorothy Rowe (author of several best-selling books about depression), 'Pneumonia is not caused by a lack of penicillin.' However, the same could be said of many of the other drugs we have discussed so far – they treat the symptoms, but do not cure the disease.

The role of psychotropic drugs in society continues to be controversial. There is evidence that 'talking treatments' – such as psychotherapy, cognitive therapy and counselling – are effective in treating mental illnesses.

The evidence comparing cognitive therapy with drugs for depression is equally impressive. In cognitive therapy – which is shorter in duration than conventional psychotherapy – the patient is taught to challenge the negative or aberrant thought patterns or beliefs that lie at the core of their condition. There is even evidence, from positron emission tomography (PET) scanning (a technique which allows the study of the chemical functioning of the brain) that cognitive therapy for obsessive compulsive disorder (OCD) produces changes in the brain similar to those observed after drug therapy.

There are some mental health professionals who would like to see the use of drugs in psychiatry dropped altogether. Chief among these is Peter Breggin, author of *Toxic Psychiatry* (which is as hard on the profession as the title suggests), himself a psychiatrist of many years standing who relies almost completely on talking treatments for his patients.

On the other hand, there are doctors and scientists who think the use of psychotropic drugs should be extended to enhance the mental functioning and well-being of supposedly 'normal' individuals. This vision is known as cosmetic pharmacology, and includes the potential use of drugs such as memory enhancers. Some doctors already use the anti-depressant Prozac in this way to help build self-esteem in patients with no obvious mental disorder. As we start to understand more about neuroscience, surely such opportunities for cosmetic pharmacology will increase. Drug companies are, understandably, always on the lookout for new markets. With an ageing population, there may be a demand for drugs that can keep mental functioning – such as memory and learning – sharp into later life. And with an increasing emphasis on quality of life among the population, maybe people will be unwilling to put up with minor personality defects, such as shyness, if these can readily be fixed by a drug that acts on the brain in a very specific way.

The chemical brain

The brain is composed of at least 100 billion neurons, whose job it is to transmit information from body to brain, and back again – or maybe just between different parts of the brain. If being human can be reduced to physiology, then neuronal transmission accounts for not just the machine-like activities of the body, such as movement, but also for the higher functions including memory, learning, emotion, thought and creativity.

A neuron has three main parts (Fig. 8.1). It has a cell body, with a nucleus and all the other apparatus of a typical cell. Then there are projections called dendrites (the word comes from the Greek word *dendros*, meaning 'tree') which carry information to the cell body. The longer projection (those going down the spinal cord may be up to four feet (120 cm) long) is called the axon, and these carry information *away from* the cell body. Dendrites and axons are sometimes also called nerve fibres.

The way information is carried from one neuron to another is electro-chemical in nature. A 'resting' neuron (i.e. not carrying information) is electrically negative compared to its exterior, with the concentration of positive sodium ions being higher on the outside. In this state, the cell is said to be polarised – because there is a big charge difference between the inside and the outside.

But if an electrical impulse arises within the cell body, or dendrite – as a result of information conveyed by a neighbouring neuron – then the charge difference between the interior and exterior of the cell decreases and the cell becomes depolarised. The cell membrane suddenly becomes more permeable to sodium ions, which rush in, triggering a wave of electrical activity down the axon which is equivalent to the transmission of an electrical impulse (Fig. 8.1).

What happens when the impulse reaches the end of the axon though? At one time, it was thought that the network of neurons in the brain was continuous, like a national railway system. Then the Nobel Prize-winning Spanish neuroanatomist Santiago Ramón y Cajal (1852–1934) showed that there was a distinct gap – later called a synapse – between the axon terminus of one cell and the next neuron. Later research showed that the electrical

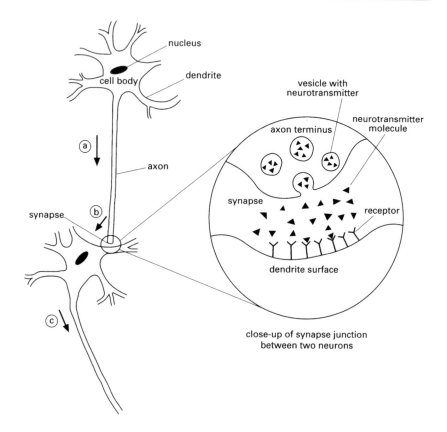

Fig. 8.1. Transmission across a synapse. Two neurons are shown on the left-hand side of the diagram, with the direction of transmission of information shown by arrows. An electrical impulse passes down the axon of the top neuron (a), triggering the release of neurotransmitter across the synapse (b), which causes an electrical impulse to travel through the dendrite, cell body and axon of the lower neuron (c). A close-up of the neuron is shown to the right-hand side of the figure. The electrical impulse causes excitatory neurotransmitter molecules to spill out of their vesicles into the synapse. They dock onto specific receptor molecules on the dendritic surface of the second neuron, causing that neuron to fire as they do so.

impulse does not leap, as a spark, across the synapse. Instead it stimulates the release of chemicals called neurotransmitters, which convey the message in chemical form from one neuron to another.

The neurotransmitter is usually released from tiny 'packets' called vesicles in the axon terminus. The molecules move through the synapse and lock onto specific receptors in the neighbouring neurons (Fig. 8.1). There may be more than one type of receptor for a particular neurotransmitter, occuring in different parts of the brain – a finding that has important implications for drug design, as we shall see.

Once the neurotransmitter has locked onto the receptor and so conveyed its message to the receiving neuron, it is either transported back to the originating neuron, where it is re-absorbed (by the so-called re-uptake mechanism) or is broken down by enzymes in the synapse.

Around 45 different neurotransmitters have been identified within the brain. Researchers believe there could be many more. Some excite the receiving neuron – that is, they send the message on – while others are inhibitory, keeping their receiving neuron in a resting state. Different neurotransmitters 'map' onto different brain functions, and often they are involved in more than one function. For instance, dopamine is involved in both movement and emotion, while serotonin appears to govern many different functions from aggression and appetite to the action of the heart.

Each of the neurotransmitters is a target – or potential target – for psychotropic drugs. Those in common use act in most of the ways already described in Chapter 1 – that is, they act on neurotransmitter receptors, or they inhibit enzymes involved in the breakdown of the neurotransmitter or they block its re-uptake. The resulting alteration in neurotransmitter concentration within the synapse may have a profound effect upon brain function.

Mending the mind? Drugs and mental illness

Before the discovery of psychotropic drugs in the 1950s and 1960s, the outlook for people suffering from mental illness was truly bleak. There were only three types of treatment available – electroconvulsive therapy (ECT), insulin coma, and psychosurgery. As a result many patients spent their entire lives imprisoned in large mental institutions. Others fell victim to the 'revolving door' – once outside hospital they could not cope, became ill again, and were rapidly re-admitted.

In ECT electrodes are placed on the temples and a shock passed through the brain, causing a convulsion. How it works is unknown, but it can relieve very severe depression (for which it is still used today, albeit in a more refined version). In the past, ECT was used quite indiscriminately for all manner of mental conditions including schizophrenia. ECT can have quite severe side effects on the memory; it often wipes out memories of pre-treatment events and may interfere with learning after the treatment.

Insulin coma was used as a treatment for schizophrenia and involved giving the patient large doses of insulin until they became unconscious (because of the dramatic fall in blood sugar), and remained so for several days. It has no therapeutic effect (although it obviously quietens noisy patients) and has long fallen into disuse.

Psychosurgery involves a process called leucotomy, in which various pathways within the brain are interrupted by cutting nerve fibres. The commonest procedure was lobotomy (or prefrontal leucotomy) which severed the connection between the thalamus and the frontal lobe. The thalamus, which lies deep in the brain, relays sensory data to the cerebral cortex while the frontal lobe is associated with personality, judgement and other higher functions. Disconnecting the two was said to calm severe emotional tension, although it often also caused severe brain dysfunction. Like ECT, it was used as a cure-all. And like ECT it is still used today – although the procedure is far more sophisticated – in cases that have failed to respond to any other form of treatment.

On the whole, however, these treatments have been replaced by modern drug therapies. The days of the long-stay mental hospital are over and most patients with mental illness now live in the community. However, 'care in the community' has not been an unqualified success. Drugs have undoubtedly played a major part in making it possible – but most people with mental illness need more than drugs to enable them to live happy and productive lives, such as decent housing, and social support. These other resources have not always been forthcoming.

Drugs, dopamine and schizophrenia

The two mental conditions on which drug therapy has had the most impact are schizophrenia and depression. Schizophrenia is characterised by disordered thought – for instance, sufferers may say that their thoughts are being broadcast, or are being inserted into their minds by an external agency. Auditory hallucinations are common; schizophrenics often hear angry, hostile, accusing voices discussing them in the third person. They may also have delusions – false beliefs that they are someone they are not (like Jesus Christ) or that people are persecuting them. Such symptoms are said to be psychotic; they indicate that the patient has lost touch with reality. Schizophrenia is also characterised by a number of so-called negative symptoms such as social withdrawal, lack of drive and motivation, and self-neglect – all of which make it difficult to function in society.

Schizophrenia usually strikes in young adulthood and affects one per cent of the population. It is a very old disease and so cannot be blamed on the stresses of modern life. Looking back, psychiatrists have suggested that Nebuchadnezzar in the Old Testament and Saint Theresa of Avila were both schizophrenics. Left untreated, perhaps one-quarter of people with schizophrenia will recover spontaneously – the rest will go through life with some degree of impairment. One in ten commits suicide.

The cause of schizophrenia remains unknown, although many theories have been put forward. There is a strong genetic component – although the genes responsible have not been identified. However, the child of a schizophrenic has a 10 per cent chance of developing the disease, while an identical twin has a 50 per cent chance. (Identical twins share the same genes and the frequency of a disease in a twin compared to its frequency in the general population gives some idea of the importance of genetic factors.) This points to an inherited biochemical defect – something that could be a drug target.

That parental, social and environmental factors are also important is undeniable. In the 1960s, the theories of British psychiatrist Ronnie Laing – which, put simply, suggested that schizophrenia was an understandable response to bad parenting – were much in vogue and still influence mental health workers today. However, most researchers today are looking for defective brain chemistry, or subtle brain lesions, when they probe for the causes of schizophrenia.

The development of drugs for schizophrenia has done much to advance this search for the cause of the disease. As with many of the other drugs discussed so far, the first drug for schizophrenia was discovered accidentally by the French neurosurgeon Henri Laborit, who was looking for something to sedate patients before surgery. He first tried an antihistamine called pro-methazine, which was already noted for its sedating properties. Histamine is a chemical which the body releases as part of its inflammatory response – either to genuine injuries or pathogens, or to allergic triggers of asthma and hay fever. It causes swelling, pain, redness, a runny nose and watery eyes – hence, antihistamines are useful for treating the symptoms of hay fever. Promethazine worked well for Laborit's patients so he went on to try other antihistamines to 'fine-tune' the clinical response. He was so impressed with a related compound called chlorpromazine that he recommended it to his psychiatric colleagues for calming their patients. It worked like a dream – at least as far as the doctors were concerned – on hyperactive, manic and deluded patients. Many, but not all, were suffering from schizophrenia.

Before long chlorpromazine – or Largactil (Thorazine in the US) – was being used in mental hospitals all over Europe and the USA. Shortly afterwards began the long exodus of patients from these institutions. Even if they were not cured, they were certainly better behaved and stood a better chance of making their way in life.

However, there has been much criticism of Largactil and its use in prisons and old people's homes to 'manage' difficult people. Some have described it as a 'chemical cosh'. There is little doubt that Largactil has been – and probably is – used in this way. However, early clinical studies suggested that it does have a genuine anti-schizophrenic effect over and above that of sedation. Patients on barbiturates – a pure sedative – were compared with those on chlorpromazine. The latter group showed clear improvements in the thought disorders that are so characteristic of schizophrenia, compared to the barbiturate group.

This was important. If researchers discovered just what chlorpromazine was 'correcting' in the brain, then they would have an important pointer to what actually goes wrong in schizophrenia. The techniques for probing the action of chlorpromazine in the brain (which are applicable, by the way, to studies of other drugs on the brain) were developed by many scientists, prominent among whom is Solomon Snyder of Johns Hopkins Medical School in Baltimore. Typically, an animal would be injected with neurotransmitter bearing a radioactive 'tag'. This would bind to its receptor in the brain. After killing the animal, slices of brain tissue can be exposed to photographic emulsion (which 'fogs' when it is exposed to radioactivity). This creates an image of neurotransmitter–receptor binding which can be studied under the microscope (the technique was used by Snyder and his team to locate opiate receptors in the brain).

If radioactive dopamine is used in such an experiment, it can be shown that drugs such as chlorpromazine tend to knock it off its receptor; there is less radioactivity in tissue samples from animals treated with the drugs because less dopamine can bind to the receptor. So the neuroleptics (the clinical term for chlorpromazine and other anti-schizophrenic drugs – sometimes also called major tranquillisers) appear to act by blocking dopamine receptors. There are now over 20 neuroleptics in clinical use. The phenothiazines are related chemically to chlorpromazine. Another major group is the butyrophenones, of which haloperidol is probably the most potent neuroleptic in clinical use. More recently, the thioxanthenes, of which flup-enthixol is the main example, have been developed.

All these chemically diverse neuroleptics block two subtypes of dopamine receptor called D_1 and D_2 – leaving the other subtypes (there are at least four in all) alone. This action – especially at D_2 – is responsible for the anti-psychotic effects of these drugs. It has led to the theory that schizophrenia arises from an over-activity of dopamine in the brain (which is almost certainly an over-simplification).

D_2 receptors occur in an area of the brainstem, called the tegmentum, on neurons extending into the limbic region, which is concerned with the regulation of emotion. It is thought that over-activity of this pathway some-how leads to the thought disorder of schizophrenia, and neuroleptics exert their anti-psychotic effects by modulating this. Seventy per cent of schizophrenics respond to drugs. The problem is that the neuroleptics do not cure schizophrenia – they merely deal with the symptoms and once a patient stops taking them relapse is almost certain.

Many people find it hard to commit to taking drugs long-term. It is even harder to persuade psychotic patients to keep to a drug schedule when they lack insight into their condition – and doubly difficult when the drugs have serious side effects. For there is also a high concentration of dopamine and D_2 receptors in a tiny area of the brain stem called the substantia nigra (so-called because the cells contain the dark pigment melanin). These neurons extend to an area called the corpus striatum, the part of the brain responsible for the co-ordination of limb movement. People suffering from Parkinson's disease are deficient in dopamine and this particular pathway is affected – leading to rigidity, tremor, spasm, and sudden jerky movements. Around 75 per cent of people on neuroleptics suffer the same symptoms – which is hardly conducive to trying to live a normal life while also coping with schizophrenia. Worse, another syndrome known as tardive dyskinesia starts up after prolonged treatment. Tardive dyskinesia is characterised by sudden jerky movements of the tongue, mouth, arms and legs. It appears to come from an increase in the number of dopamine receptors in response to their long-term blockade by neuroleptics. It is as if the drug has overshot the mark in its attempt to regulate the dopamine pathways.

All this represents a significant challenge to the pharmaceutical industry. The first response was to formulate neuroleptics as a long-acting ('depot') injection to get around the problem of non-compliance with tablets. However, this does not address the problem of side effects – which requires new insights into brain chemistry.

So the last few years has seen more attention given to developing 'cleaner' neuroleptics. Ideally one would want a D_2 antagonist that only acted on the dopamine pathway involving the limbic system. A new class of drug, the benzamides, partly fills this requirement – having significantly fewer Parkinsonian side effects. But perhaps the greatest breakthrough in neuroleptics in recent years has been clozapine (Clozaril). First brought onto the market in the late 1960s, it soon acquired a bad reputation because it causes aplastic anaemia in around one per cent of patients, depleting the body of white blood cells needed to fight infection.

But then it was shown that patients who had not responded to other neuroleptics did respond to clozapine. Moreover, clozapine was different in that it seemed to tackle the negative symptoms of schizophrenia – giving the patient a far better shot at a normal life. Better still, it is relatively free of Parkinsonian effects, which led researchers to believe that it could be acting somewhere other than at the D_2 receptors. The current thinking is that clozapine may also block another neurotransmitter, serotonin (of which more later), which could also account for its anti-psychotic effects.

Clozapine seems to give hope where before there was none. There are many case reports of lives being transformed by the drug. But, without regular blood checks, clozapine could be fatal. It is also expensive, compared to other neuroleptics. There is a newer drug, risperidone, which is free of the risk of aplastic anaemia, and acts much like clozapine – although it does give rise to more side effects. And there are several more drugs for this debilitating illness in the pipeline.

The anti-depressant revolution

Depression is the other major mental illness. Said to affect one in 20 of the population at any one time, depression comes in many different forms – from a persistent feeling of discouragement to full-blown psychosis complete with delusions and hallucinations. Where depression alternates with periods of over-activity known as mania it is known as manic depression – a condition which affects about one per cent of the population. As with schizophrenia, there is a genetic component to depression – and particularly with manic depression.

An interesting difference between schizophrenia and depression is that the latter does not always sap talent, creativity and motivation. Some of the world's greatest artists and thinkers have suffered from depression in some form or another – Virginia Woolf, Leo Tolstoy, Gerald Manley Hopkins and Robert Schumann. Better still, some – such as Pulitzer Prize winner William Styron – have written movingly about their experience of the condition, which has undoubtedly led to greater public recognition and understanding of the suffering involved.

There is no blood test or other physical test for depression (not yet anyway) so doctors have to rely upon a checklist of typical symptoms – such as waking early, feelings of guilt and worthlessness, lack of appetite – to make the diagnosis. The condition may arise in response to an external event such as bereavement, illness or redundancy, or there may be no apparent cause.

There are a number of biochemical theories on how depression arises – these have developed alongside clinical studies of anti-depressant drugs over the last 30 years or so. Chief among these is the biogenic amine theory which suggests that mood depends upon the levels of specific neurotransmitters in the brain. The three neurotransmitters involved are dopamine – which we have already met – noradrenaline, and serotonin. All are amines (a specific group of compounds containing a nitrogen atom) and are called biogenic because they arise within the body.

Coincidentally, the first anti-depressant drug was discovered around the same time as the first neuroleptic. Iproniazid started out as an anti-tuberculosis drug in 1952. Before long doctors noticed that patients on iproniazid seemed remarkably cheerful and the drug was launched as a treatment for depression in 1957. Four hundred thousand patients took it – before the incidence of severe side effects led to its withdrawal.

However, iproniazid was rapidly followed by a new anti-depressant called imipramine, which is still in use today. Imipramine is one of a group of anti-depressants known as the tricyclics. Research showed that the tricyclics work by slowing the re-uptake of both noradrenaline and serotonin, thereby effectively increasing their concentrations in the synapses. Imipramine has an overall stimulant effect and is good for depressed patients whose chief symptoms are apathy, lethargy, and exhaustion. A related compound, amitriptyline, has a more sedating effect and would be more helpful for patients who are anxious, agitated and suffer insomnia.

Because the noradrenaline and serotonin act in several parts of the brain, and also in other parts of the body, the older tricyclics are relatively 'dirty' drugs giving rise to many side effects. For instance, noradrenaline is also the body's 'flight or fight' hormone and increasing its concentration leads to physiological arousal – so sweating and a dry mouth are very common in patients on tricyclics. The dry mouth can even lead to tooth decay, for it encourages infection. Dizziness is another common side effect, which could interfere with driving or operating machinery.

Newer tricyclics such as desimipramine and dothiepin act more specifically upon noradrenaline and are said to be very effective. Lofepramine, also fairly recent, is associated with fewer side effects than the other tricyclics.

A second category of anti-depressants is the monoamine oxidase inhibitors (MAOIs). Monoamine oxidase is the enzyme which breaks down biogenic amines. If this is inhibited then levels of the amines will increase. Unfortunately, some foodstuffs – such as cheese and red wine – contain an amine called tyramine which is also broken down by monoamine oxidase in the gut and liver. Otherwise tyramine may cause a dangerous increase in blood pressure which could lead to a stroke. MAOIs also inhibit the gut and liver enzymes, so patients on these anti-depressants need to avoid tyramine-containing foods in their diet. This is a major drawback; depressed patients are forgetful and may fail to register these directions. Worse, if they are suicidal, then they have just been handed the means of committing the act on impulse. Traditionally MAOIs have not been much used – except where tricyclics proved ineffective. However, they are now being more widely prescribed because of the discovery that they are quite effective in the treatment of eating disorders, panic disorder, and phobias. There is also a new MAOI on the market called moclobemide which leaves the gut and liver enzymes alone, eliminating the need for dietary restrictions.

Around 60–70 per cent of depressed patients respond to tricyclics or MAOIs the first time round. If the first drug does not work, others can be tried – pushing the overall response rate up to over 90 per cent. This makes depression a highly treatable condition. However, anti-depressant therapy does not always work as well as it should. First, many people who could benefit do not get anti-depressants – either because they do not recognise themselves as being ill or, worse, they do not think they deserve treatment. Second, family doctors do not always recognise a depressed patient – the condition often comes 'disguised' as a physical complaint such as fatigue or stomach pain. And finally, patients are often reluctant to take anti-depressants believing (wrongly, as it happens) that they must be addictive because they act on the mind.

And even if the patient does start on an appropriate drug, there is still a problem – over and above the side effects mentioned above. For some unknown reason, most anti-depressants take several weeks to exert their full effects, while the side effects kick in almost immediately. In other words, patients can generally expect to feel worse before they feel better. Not much comfort for someone in the depths of despair. It helps if they like and trust their doctor or psychiatrist who can then persuade them to stay the course. Insomnia and anxiety tend to be the first symptoms that clear up. These improvements may be sufficient to encourage the patient to stay the course long enough to experience the full effects of the anti-depressant.

Depression tends to be a self-limiting condition and often clears up within a few weeks (although, as we shall see, it may recur and can become chronic). This, coupled with the fact that there is a strong placebo response in depression, with up to 30 per cent of patients in clinical trials responding to 'dummy' pills, has led some doctors – chiefly Peter Breggin who was mentioned above – to state that in fact anti-depressants have no therapeutic value. These sceptics attribute any beneficial effects to either a placebo response, or to the natural resolution of the illness – which would have happened anyway but coincided with the apparent clinical response a few weeks after starting anti-depressant therapy.

On the other hand, there are other doctors who advocate more widespread use of anti-depressants. Nowadays they will start treatment early, give higher doses, and keep the patient on the drug for at least six months – and perhaps even for life. Critics say this group has been brainwashed by the pharmaceutical industry, but there appear to be sound clinical reasons for stepping up the use of anti-depressants. In recent years, Robert Post of the National Institute for Mental Health in Bethesda, Maryland, has developed the so-called 'kindling' theory of depression. It has long been known that depression tends to recur – even though an individual episode may clear up relatively quickly.

Post's clinical studies have shown that while while 60 per cent of first depressive episodes were preceded by a precipitating trauma, this was true of only 30 per cent of second episodes and around 6 per cent of subsequent episodes. He noted that depression would often follow a progressive, deteriorating course, with the intervals between episodes getting shorter, while the episodes themselves got longer. Worse, the episodes began to trigger themselves, for no obvious reason. Post reasoned that in some way an initial episode of depression subtly – and permanently – alters brain chemistry, rendering the individual more susceptible to repeated attacks. He likens this to the kindling which can set a fire alight.

The kindling phenomenon is particularly noticeable in manic-depressive disorder. Over the years the manic episodes become wilder, the depressions more suicidal and the trauma suffered by the individual and his family harder to deal with. The kindling theory may also go some way to explaining why late-onset depression (with the first episode occurring after the age of 60) tends to be more severe, with higher risk of suicide and more hypochondriacal features. It may be that the stresses and strains of everyday life gradually alter the brain's chemistry, making it more vulnerable to the slightest trauma.

A tragic example is the suicide of writer and chemist Primo Levi in 1987, over 40 years after surviving World War II in a concentration camp. Is it possible that that early trauma was represented as a slow-acting poison in the brain, whose toxic effects were only realised after many years? One candidate for this brain toxin is the stress hormone cortisol, which is produced by the adrenal glands just above the kidneys. It has long been known that cortisol levels remain high for years after an episode of depression, and the adrenal glands are often enlarged in suicides, suggesting abnormal secretion of the hormone. Recent studies from a team at Washington State University suggest that high cortisol may also affect the brain – specifically by shrinking the hippocampus, the area concerned with learning and memory.

It is too soon to tell whether lifelong treatment with anti-depressants can alter the course of events, but psychiatrists and patients alike are increasingly taking this option. Incidentally, for manic depressive patients this usually means lithium and perhaps the anti-convulsant drug carbamazepine, rather than an anti-depressant. Lithium, in the form of a simple chemical salt, appears to work by replacing some of the excess sodium in the brain cells of patients during a manic episode.

The other reason why the use of anti-depressants is on the increase is the development of a third category of drugs – the selective serotonin re-uptake inhibitors (SSRIs), of which fluoxetine (Prozac) is the best-known example. Unlike other anti-depressants, the SSRIs act only on serotonin. Blocking its re-uptake into the neurons from which it was released increases its concentration in the synapses. This specific effect on just one neurotransmitter makes the SSRI's 'cleaner' drugs than most of the tricyclics and the MAOIs.

The SSRIs are no more effective in relieving depression than other drugs, and still have that annoying time lag before the therapeutic effects set in. But they are in a class of their own because they are relatively free of side effects. This means that they are increasingly used upon less 'ill' patients (for whom a doctor may hesitate to prescribe a drug with significant side effects). Prozac, and related compounds, are used for a range of conditions related to depression such as obsessive-compulsive disorder, panic anxiety, eating disorders, pre-menstrual syndrome and substance abuse. It also tends to reduce alcohol consumption. No wonder Prozac is fourth in the top 20 best selling drugs (see Table 1).

Serotonin, like the other neurotransmitters we have discussed, has multiple roles. It is involved in sleep–wake cycles, appetite (some of the slimming drugs discussed in Chapter 5 work on serotonin pathways) and in emotion. Specifically serotonin is involved in impulse control and feelings of comfort, self-esteem and security.

Many studies have shown that low status, aggression and anti-social behaviour are associated with low serotonin levels. For instance, Michael McGuire of the University of California has shown that in vervet monkeys the dominant male has 50 per cent more serotonin in his blood than other monkeys. After a struggle in which dominance was swapped from one monkey to another, serotonin levels increased in the newly dominant monkey, and fell in the recently dominant animal to 50 per cent below the average subordinate male. This suggests that social status influences serotonin levels. But could serotonin influence social status? Yes – in the monkey experiments, animals given Prozac tend to become dominant, suggesting that serotonin may act as a chemical 'drive to success'.

But how does all this translate to humans? A study of American servicemen from the 1970s showed that the most violent recruits had the lowest serotonin. So did prisoners who were most likely to re-offend. Children who torture animals and who are hostile to their parents have low serotonin. And serotonin levels have even been used to predict which of a group of 8–10 year-olds would be the most aggressive two years later. These links between low serotonin and anti-social behaviour have led some psychiatrists to describe serotonin as having a 'policing' function within the brain. Not only does it put the brakes on anti-social behaviour, it also creates a feeling of confidence and security which acts as a basis for achieving high status and success.

While no one is openly advocating the mass medication of delinquents with SSRIs, there is fascinating testimony of what can happen if near-normal people are given Prozac – chiefly from Peter Kramer, author of *Listening to Prozac: Antidepressants and the Remaking of the Self*. According to Kramer, Prozac can 'remodel' the personality – creating confidence and self-esteem. In the therapeutic sense, it can make a patient more receptive to psychotherapy – or even achieve the same results as years of patient committment to psychotherapy on the part of the patient and the therapist. In a very real sense, it appears to alter personality.

All this appears to bring us close to the concept of 'cosmetic pharmacology' (although Kramer does not actually advocate this). If the brain chemistry underpinning personality could be worked out, then it might be possible to develop drugs to fine-tune the chemistry to create the personality of one's choice. It may sound absurdly simplistic (to say nothing of having sinister 'Brave New World' overtones) – but in fact US psychiatrist Robert Cloninger has already begun developing a neurochemical theory of personality. It sounds like a throwback to the old idea of the four bodily 'humours' – where a person rich in 'choleric' would be aggressive, and those with lots of 'black bile' were melancholic and so on. However, at least Cloninger's three 'neurohumours' actually exist – and they are dopamine, noradrenaline, and serotonin.

According to Cloninger's theory noradrenaline levels are associated with rejection sensitivity (shyness, and worrying what people think about you, in simpler language). Serotonin is associated with harm avoidance (comfort and security), while dopamine correlates with stimulus-seeking behaviour. Cloninger would use the three neurotransmitters as three independent axes – describing personality according to a person's level of the three substances (in the same way as you might locate a point in space according to its co-ordinates on Cartesian x, y and z axes). To modify personality on this basis, you would just have to take a drug to alter your levels of serotonin, noradrenaline, or dopamine. No one is working on this – but some of Kramer's clinical studies on Prozac appear to be taking a step in the direction of remodelling the personality.

The SSRIs are in a class of their own – and Prozac in particular has been the subject of what is probably excessive media attention. There was bound to be a backlash, and it came in the form of the Joe Wesbecker case. On September 14 1989, 47-year-old Joseph Wesbecker of Louisville, Kentucky returned to the printing works where he had been employed for many years (he was on sick leave) and shot 20 of his co-workers, killing eight of them, before turning the gun on himself.

Wesbecker had a long history of mental illness and had been prescribed many different drugs. But shortly before the killings, he had been put on Prozac. It seemed to make him agitated – so much so that a case was brought against Eli Lilly, Prozac's manufacturers, five years later by the survivors of the massacre. They seemed to have a strong case. In 1990 Martin Teicher of Harvard Medical School had reported six patients who had become intensely suicidal on Prozac. Other reports suggested that Prozac could make people violent.

This sounds paradoxical. Prozac is meant to enhance serotonin levels, and that should make people *less* violent. It was possible, argued the prosecution, that the brain might respond to an 'artificial' increase in serotonin by turning down production in an attempt to maintain the status quo. Which, say critics of psychotropic drugs, only illustrates the dangers of tampering with something as complex as the chemistry of the brain. Unfortunately, this issue was never properly aired in the Wesbecker case – because Eli Lilly made a secret deal with the plaintiffs.

The Wesbecker case may have made some psychiatrists pause for thought before they prescribe Prozac to potentially suicidal patients. However, an analysis of all the reports on Prozac and suicide showed the risks were more apparent than real (although, it has to be said, the work was done by scientists working for the manufacturers of the drug).

Prozac, and other anti-depressants, are more popular than ever. Not just for the reasons already discussed but because they are also filling the vacuum left by the decline in prescribing of tranquillisers. Indeed, some psychiatrists now believe that anxiety (formerly treated with tranquillisers) is just another form of depression.

The rise and fall of tranquillisers

Most tranquillisers belong to the chemical category called the benzodiazepines. The best-known examples are Valium (diazepam) and Librium (chlordiazepoxide). They were introduced into Britain in the early 1960s and were to become among the most widely prescribed drugs of all time. By 1979, one in five women and one in ten men were on benzodiazepines for a wide range of problems from fear of the dentist to exam nerves – as well as for more chronic anxiety problems. Related drugs were developed – such as alprazolam (Xanax), which was prescribed for panic anxiety, and triazolam (Halcion), a short-acting benzodiazepine widely used as a sleeping drug.

The benzodiazepines more or less replaced barbiturates, which had been in widespread use since the 1920s, and were thought to be far safer. Barbiturates are extremely addictive and can be lethal in overdose – especially with alcohol. They have been responsible for numerous suicides and accidental deaths.

Benzodiazepines are both anxiolytic (relieving anxiety) and hypnotic (sleep inducing). They work by enhancing the action of the inhibitory neurotransmitter gamma-aminobutyric acid (GABA), and so quieten neural activity, producing a sedating effect. In 1977 researchers in Denmark and Switzerland, working independently, discovered benzodiazepine receptors in brain tissue. This was – and is – a bit of a puzzle. People are not born with Valium in them, so where is the natural substance that binds to these receptors? There must be a molecule in the brain which is a natural benzodi-azepine – in the same way that endorphins are a natural form of morphine (binding to μ opioid receptors) – but so far it has not been discovered.

Further research showed that the benzodiazepine receptors were located mainly (but not exclusively) in the limbic system, which deals with the regulation of emotional states. They are especially concentrated in the amygdala, an almond-shaped structure within the limbic system, and prob-ably form neural circuits which help modify the experience of fear. It turns out that the GABA and benzodiazepine receptors both occupy different sites on the same large protein molecule. When Valium or another tranquilliser molecule binds its receptor, it subtly alters the shape of this protein in such a way as to allow stronger binding of GABA. The result is the quietening effect referred to earlier.

Barbiturates and alcohol both bind to a third site on this receptor, and also enhance GABA's action. Now we know why the combination of bar-biturates and alcohol, or even benzodiazepines and alcohol, is so dangerous. There are GABA–benzodiazepine–barbiturate receptors elsewhere in the brain, such as the brain stem and the cerebral cortex. Alcohol and tranquil-lisers together greatly enhance GABA's inhibitory effect on the brain so that vital neural circuits involved in maintaining breathing and heartbeat close down altogether.

Besides the dangers of combining them with alcohol, the main problem with benzodiazepines is that they cause physiological and psychological dependence. If people stop taking them after long-term use they suffer a range of unpleasant symptoms such as 'rebound' anxiety, insomnia, shaking and palpitations. To relieve this discomfort they will often resort to taking the drug again – hence appearing to be 'hooked' on it.

These days a responsible doctor will only prescribe benzodiazepines when strictly necessary – in periods of extreme stress, for example, or to give someone a decent night's sleep when they really need it. No one should be on benzodiazepines for more than a month at a time – although there is evidence that a minority of people are still taking them long-term. This is especially worrying in older people who are more prone to the sedating effects of tranquillisers and may be more likely to have falls and other accidents while taking them. There is also concern that the 'hangover' effect of benzodiazepine hypnotics may be responsible for a number of otherwise inexplicable road accidents.

Halcion, which had become the world's most frequently prescribed hypnotic, was banned in the UK in 1991 because of concerns about side effects such as daytime anxiety, panic attacks and even delusions. Even so, Halcion is still prescribed in many other countries, and some doctors think it is still a very useful drug. And the sale of temazepam, usually the drug of choice for insomnia in the UK, has had to be restricted because of evidence of its abuse.

People on long-term benzodiazepines need to withdraw from them gradually under medical supervision. And they may still need an alternative method for dealing with their anxiety and/or insomnia. Although it is often said that lack of sleep never killed anyone, both anxiety and insomnia if left untreated may lead to alcoholism, depression and even suicide. Buspirone, a serotonin antagonist, is said to be relatively free of side effects, and does not cause dependence. And the beta blockers – which have already been discussed in Chapter 5 – are useful for treating the physical symptoms of anxiety such as trembling and palpitations.

There are also new non-benzodiazepine hypnotics, such as zopiclone (Zimovane) and diphenhydramine (Nytol). The latter is actually an old antihistamine. As a hypnotic, it exploits the sedating effects of this group of compounds which are so annoying when they are used for hay fever and other allergies.

Insomnia and anxiety often resolve themselves without drug treatment. Where they do not, and given that drug treatments are not suitable in the long term, other solutions must be looked for. In the case of insomnia, simple 'sleep hygiene' measures often do the trick. Getting up at the same time each morning – even at weekends – avoiding alcohol, heavy meals and caffeine before bed, and sleeping in comfort can work wonders. And for anxiety, there are many non-drug therapies – relaxation, massage, yoga and aromatherapy to name but a few. In many cases, psychotherapy or counselling may be the best way of resolving issues that give rise to chronic anxiety.

All this is not to say that benzodiazepines no longer have any use. An injection of Valium before surgery (the 'pre-med') is very useful in helping patients relax physically and mentally before anaesthetic gases are applied through a mask.

Medicating naughty children – the puzzle of attention deficit disorder (ADD)

Restlessness and impulsive naughty behaviour might sound like part and parcel of childhood, adolescence and growing up. But increasingly, in the eyes of some psychiatrists, teachers, and parents, this kind of behaviour is seen as abnormal and is labelled as attention deficit disorder (ADD). There is no biological test for ADD, although brain scans have shown lesions in the areas associated with impulse control.

It may be tempting to suppose that ADD is a modern condition, associated with environmental pollution or junk food (such as fish fingers, squash and snacks containing the orange food colouring tartrazine which some children are sensitive to). However, there have also been suggestions that ADD is a very old – albeit unrecognised – disorder, which afflicted illustrious people such as Leonardo da Vinci and Winston Churchill.

Children with ADD are a pest in the classroom (if they can stay there for any length of time). They annoy the teacher and their fellow classmates and, worst of all, they do not learn anything because they cannot sit still for long enough to benefit from a lesson. Increasingly ADD is being treated with a drug called Ritalin – particularly in the US where between three and ten per cent of children take it. Ritalin is also widely used in Canada and Australia. In the UK, take-up has been slower, with only around 6000 children taking it at the present time.

Surprisingly, perhaps, Ritalin is a stimulant which increases dopamine concentration (one school of thought suggests that ADD arises from a defect in dopamine receptors, leading to lowered dopamine activity). On Ritalin, children's attention span increases sufficiently for them to be able to start learning.

Needless to say, the whole issue of Ritalin and ADD is hugely controversial. The very existence of ADD as a clinical condition is questioned by those who blame poor teaching, poor parenting and adverse environmental conditions for children's learning difficulties. And the prospect of mass-medicating young children with drugs that affect the brain – maybe for years – is intrinsically worrying. An EEG (electroencephalagram) test of ADD is promised soon; maybe this will clear up some of the doubt and uncertainty surrounding the condition. If there turns out to be no definite diagnosis – or brain lesion – then the experts could start to tackle the genuine causes of learning difficulties. On the other hand, if a specific physiological 'marker' is found, it could lead to better understanding and treatment of the disorder.

When the brain dies before the body – the challenge of Alzheimer's disease

The mental illnesses discussed above are thought to be rooted in the chemistry of the brain (although there is mounting evidence that anatomical lesions may also be involved; scans have shown shrinkage of the hippocampus, a brain structure involved in memory, in chronic depression, for instance). In contrast, there are also mental disorders which are associated with specific brain damage caused by tumours, strokes, toxins such as excess alcohol and other factors. As far as drug therapy is concerned, Alzheimer's disease is probably the most important – because it is relatively common and has been the subject of intensive basic and pharmaceutical research in recent years.

Alzheimer's disease was first described by the German physiologist Alois Alzheimer in the early years of this century. It is the commonest cause of dementia, a progressive loss of the higher brain functions such as memory, judgement, and language skills. At the same time there is a distressing deterioration of personality, often accompanied by violent outbursts and an inability to recognise friends and family. Alzheimer's disease is not, in itself, fatal – but the patient's inability to take care of himself usually leads to death within five years or so of diagnosis, even with expert care. The intervening years can impose an immense emotional, physical and financial burden on the patient's family. As one carer put it, 'it is as if the brain died before the body.' Alzheimer's is a disease of older people (although it can strike people in their 40s). It affects one per cent of people in the 60–65 age group, and between 30 and 50 per cent of the over-85s.

There are two kinds of characteristic lesions found in the post-mortem brains of Alzheimer's patients. First, there are deposits known as plaques containing a protein called β-amyloid. This is an abnormal form of a protein of unknown function called amyloid precursor protein (APP), which occurs naturally in the body. Second, there are tangles within some neurons which contain paired helical filaments consisting of an abnormal form of another brain protein called τ protein. Normal τ helps maintain the inner skeleton of the cell – a network of protein-based tubules. In its abnormal form, the skeleton collapses, forming the tangles. These two kinds of lesion lead to actual loss of functioning neurons.

There is also an associated biochemical defect. People with Alzheimer's have low levels of the neurotransmitter acetylcholine in their brains, and of the enzyme that catalyses its formation from its precursor molecule, choline. Acetylcholine, which was the first neurotransmitter to be discovered in 1921 by the German pharmacologist Otto Loewi, acts on the neuromuscular junction – that is, the synapse where a motor neuron interacts with a muscle fibre. Release of acetylcholine causes the muscle to contract. Once released, the acetylcholine is then rapidly broken down by the enzyme acetylcholinesterase.

Acetylcholine is present in all members of the animal kingdom, including insects. Many insecticides are acetylcholinesterase inhibitors; they cause a toxic build-up of acetylcholine in the insect's body. Such compounds have also been used for chemical warfare. They act as nerve gases, paralysing the breathing mechanism.

Acetylcholine-containing neurons also occur in the brain – particularly in an area known as the basal nucleus, as well as in the hippocampus, and in the cerebral cortex. Those in the first two structures are thought to play a role in laying down memories, while those in the cerebral cortex are probably associated with rational thinking. So it is no surprise to learn that the brains of Alzheimer's patients are severely depleted of acetylcholine neurons, particularly in the basal nucleus.

The cause of Alzheimer's disease remains unknown. In some cases, there is a genetic factor at work – particularly in early-onset cases. And brain damage (such as that suffered by boxers) strongly predisposes to the development of Alzheimer's, as does Down's syndrome. (The latter observation only became apparent as a result of more Down's babies surviving to adulthood.) There is no way of reversing the brain damage of Alzheimer's and therefore no cure. Acetylcholinesterase is an obvious drug target. Aricept (donepezil), the only drug on the market for Alzheimer's in the UK, is an acetylcholinesterase inhibitor, as is another drug, tacrine (Cognex) which is licensed in the US. These drugs slow down the progression of the disease, giving patients perhaps an extra year or two of extra quality of life. They cannot restore memory that has already been lost.

There are around 200 other drugs against Alzheimer's in development. One of these, Huperzine A, is derived from a traditional Chinese herbal medicine prepared from the moss *Huperzia serrata*. The remedy has long been used for confusion and schizophrenia. Scientists at the Weizmann Institute of Science in Israel have recently completed a study of the structure of Huperzine with acetylcholinesterase and think the drug could be extremely specific and so relatively free of side effects. They will also be able to use this data to try to design analogous molecules of even greater pharmacological efficacy – as described in Chapter 2.

Other drugs in development are based on nicotinic receptors in the brain, so named because they respond to nicotine as well as acetylcholine. The nicotinic receptors are thought to be especially important in learning and memory. This may explain the controversial finding that people who smoke are only about half as likely to suffer from Alzheimer's disease as non-smokers (controversial because doctors do not want to be seen to be extolling the health benefits of cigarettes; it is also hard to obtain funding for this kind of research – except from tobacco companies). It appears that smokers may have more nicotinic receptors, which therefore increases acetylcholine activity. Drugs that act on the nicotinic receptors could give the beneficial memory effects of cigarettes, without their massive drawbacks.

And then there is that old standby aspirin. Many older people have taken aspirin and other NSAIDs for many years for arthritis and related conditions. Many studies suggest that these drugs have a protective role against Alzheimer's because patients on them seem to have a lower incidence of the disease. For instance Jill Rich, and her colleagues at Johns Hopkins School of Medicine in Baltimore, studied patients who had taken NSAIDs in the previous 12 months, comparing them to patients who had not (all the patients had been diagnosed with Alzheimer's). The NSAID patients did significantly better on a whole battery of mental tests, including a naming test which is used as a marker for the disease. What is more, they also showed a slower rate of decline than the non-NSAID patients over the following year.

It is not known exactly how the NSAIDs exert their beneficial effects on cognitive functioning. The presence of specific proteins involved in the body's inflammatory response in plaques and tangles has led some researchers to wonder whether inflammation is, somehow, part and parcel of Alzheimer's. However, further experiments showed that the NSAIDs do not seem to protect from Alzheimer's by acting as anti-inflammatories. In further experiments, they did not inhibit cyclooxygenase enzyme (as discussed in Chapter 1) in the brain. Instead, aspirin and salicylic acid appear to act on glutamate, a neurotransmitter important in memory. Under certain conditions, glutamate can kill neurons (this mechanism is thought to be important in destroying brain tissue after a stroke, as discussed in Chapter 5). It triggers a cascade of biochemical activity which ends in the death of the cells by apoptosis. Aspirin appears to inhibit transcription of some of the genes involved, so damping down the cascade. There is almost certainly more to be learned about the neuroprotective aspects of aspirin, but it is good news that such a well-known and readily available drug has potential to stave off the devastation of Alzheimer's disease.

The evidence that hormone replacement therapy protects against Alzheimer's disease is mounting; this was discussed in Chapter 4.

Sharpening mental faculties – the potential of cognitive enhancers

Alongside the search for drugs to slow intellectual deterioration in Alzheimer's disease, there has been a more surreptitious search for agents that can boost mental function that is already in the normal range. There is informal use of so-called cognitive enhancers or smart drugs by many people in Europe and America, and an understated aim by some drug companies to develop similar drugs over the next ten years or so. One obvious – and vast – market is the ageing population. There is some fall-off in intellectual functioning with age (although probably not as much as some people think). This can detract from quality of life – and there is increasing emphasis on making the extra years which medical science has won for us good ones on both a mental and physical level. And younger people operating in the intellectual sphere – students, writers, and business executives, for instance – may well feel attracted towards substances that can give them an edge to cope with the increasing demands made on them.

However, the processes of memory, learning and thought are so complex (and incompletely understood) that it seems audacious to even consider drugs that would alter cognition in a controllable way. It has become increasingly apparent that many brain areas are involved in memory, which is a dynamic property of the mind encoded in shifting patterns of neuronal connections. Some of the biochemical correlates of memory have, however, been unravelled and these may be useful potential drug targets.

There are two basic kinds of memory. Procedural memory tells you how to do something, like driving a car. Declarative memory is more concerned with facts and is subdivided into semantic memory (facts such as December 25 being Christmas Day) and episodic memory (remembering what Christmas presents you got last year).

Both types of memory are laid down in a chain of biochemical and neuronal events which starts with sensory input. If animals are to be trained in a task, for instance, a wave of the neurotransmitter glutamate – the primary information carrier – is triggered within the first 15–20 minutes after exposure to the task, corresponding to the creation of short-term memory.

There is a second wave of glutamate five to eight hours later, which is associated with a surge in the production of so-called cell adhesion molecules (CAMs). As the name suggests, these molecules have 'sticky ends'. A cell adhesion molecule on one synapse can cling onto a corresponding molecule on a second synapse, allowing the creation of new neural circuits. The electrical activity – carried across the synapses by glutamate – in these new circuits is enhanced, meaning that they fire more readily to the appropriate stimuli. This strengthening of the synaptic connections is known as long-term potentiation (LTP) and is thought to be the physical form of long-term memory. The appropriate stimulus would, therefore, be some kind of memory 'trigger', such as a key word. Without LTP, response to the trigger would be muted or absent. With LTP, the full memory should come flooding back, as the appropriate neural circuits are tweaked.

There are many so-called smart drugs (or nootropics, which comes from the Greek meaning 'acting on the mind') which are thought to act on this memory mechanism. Generally these are licensed for some other use, and people will buy them by mail order from specialist companies. Of these, piracetam has actually been the subject of some respectable research; it boosts acetylcholine levels and is said to increase reading ability in dyslexics. Choline, a food supplement available in health food shops, also increases acetylcholine levels. Two other drugs, hydergine – used in the treatment of epilepsy – and propanolol, a common treatment for high blood pressure, are said to improve cognition by causing a rush of blood to the head – that is, increasing blood supply to the brain. Verapamil, and other calcium channel blockers, have also been used as smart drugs. They may work by normalising calcium flow into and out of neurons, which appears to become impaired with age.

The anti-nausea drug ondansteron (Zofran) blocks specific serotonin receptors in the brain's vomiting centres. When stimulated, these receptors appear to damp down acetylcholine levels – so blocking them may have the opposite effect. In 1990 Glaxo, ondansteron's manufacturer, began testing it as a drug for memory loss in both people suffering from Alzheimer's disease and in normal middle-aged people with Age Associated Memory Impairment. This 'new' condition can apparently be diagnosed with a memory test. Preliminary results suggest that ondansteron can reverse age-related memory decline by several years.

There is also pyroglutamate, a precursor of glutamate which is said to improve memory in both rats and elderly people – though there is no convincing evidence for a beneficial effect in younger people.

Finally, there is much excitement over a new class of compounds called ampakines which have been developed by Gary Lynch and Gary Rogers of the University of California at Irvine. Tested on normal young men they produced 20 per cent improvement in standard tests of short-term recall and learning. Men in their 60s and 70s doubled their short-term memory scores on ampakines, giving performances that rivalled those of men half their age. Now trials with Alzheimer's patients are planned.

Ampakines were developed from a drug called aniracetam which is used in Japan for memory problems. Lynch noted that aniracetam boosted LTP by stimulating a type of glutamate receptor called AMPA, thereby boosting communication within the new neural circuit. The ampakines act similarly, but their effect on LTP – shown by experiments in rats – seems to be much stronger.

A recently discovered brain protein, called CREB, could be a target for powerful new memory enhancers. Tim Tully and Jerry Yin of Cold Spring Harbor Laboratory in the US, have shown that fruit flies with enhanced levels of CREB have far better memories than flies with normal amounts. In experiments in which these flies were trained to remember an odour, they recalled it for a week – the equivalent of hundreds of years in 'human time' – after a single training session. As you might expect, flies with low levels of CREB have memories like sieves. Tully and Yin intend to develop drugs based on CREB once they have learned more about its mode of action. They see a use for these not just in boosting memory, but also wiping out distressing and troubling memories after a traumatic experience, using drugs which turn down the activity of CREB.

Drugs that work on the brain span the interface between the therapeutic and the recreational. We began by looking at how psychotropic drugs help in schizophrenia and depression and ended by considering how such drugs might enhance healthy people's cognitive abilities. Inevitably any drug that affects mood, cognition and perception will attract people for its potential to enhance the quality of their lives. We will look in greater depth at the recreational use of drugs in the next chapter.

9

Drugs of recreation and addiction

All the drugs we have considered so far are generally prescribed for medicinal purposes, and are used in a controlled way. Now we move on, to look at all those other drugs which we consume for pleasure. The use of such drugs is part of human experience around the world and is deeply rooted in our culture and history – although patterns of consumption and degrees of social and legal acceptability vary widely from drug to drug.

Most people take the caffeine in a mid-morning coffee, or the alcohol in a bottle of Sauvignon Blanc shared over dinner, for granted. What is more, there is no social stigma attached to the consumption of caffeine and the moderate use of alcohol. However, although the consumption of cannabis, Ecstasy, and cocaine is almost as widespread in some sections of society their users – if they are wise – are more discreet because of the legal restrictions surrounding these drugs. And heroin consumers are almost universally pitied because it is assumed they must have an addiction problem. Meanwhile, smokers incur increasing social disapproval with more and more restrictions being put upon public consumption of tobacco.

The legal and social restrictions on recreational drugs have a complex relationship with the pharmacological properties of each substance. Each of the drugs – even, arguably, caffeine – is habit-forming to a greater or lesser extent and therefore has the potential for inflicting harm on the individual user and on society at large. And as with prescription medicines, recreational drugs have a number of side effects. However, social, political and economic factors weigh heavily against scientific factors when it comes to formulating drug legislation. Here we will not be able to devote much space to the former – but we will review what is known of the effects of recreational drugs on the body and mind, why they give pleasure, and how that pleasure can turn to addiction.

Speeding up the body and brain: the science of stimulants

The most commonly used stimulants are caffeine, tobacco, cocaine, amphetamines and nicotine. Caffeine is the most widely consumed, the most popular, and the safest of the recreational drugs. You cannot kill yourself with caffeine-containing drinks (although you might if you injected yourself with pure caffeine). It is the main active ingredient of tea, coffee and chocolate and is found in over 100 different plant species. Why caffeine is so widely distributed in nature is not fully understood, but it may act as a pesticide. Its bitter flavour may deter insects, or it may have some undesirable effect on their nervous systems.

Caffeine-containing drinks have probably been used for many hundreds, if not thousands of years, all over the world. However, caffeine itself was not isolated until 1865. The accidental discovery of tea as a drink is often attributed to Chinese emperor Shen Nung in 2737 BC. Black tea is made from the fermented leaves of the plant *Camellia sinensis*, while green tea comes from the fresh leaves. *Camellia sinensis* is native to the Indian state of Assam and also to Myanmar (formerly known as Burma). It has long been cultivated in China is also grown today in India, Sri Lanka, and Japan.

Coffee comes mainly from the roasted and ground beans of two plants – *Coffea arabica* and *Coffea robusta*. The former is generally thought to have a finer flavour, although it contains less caffeine and is harder to grow. Coffee plants are native to Ethiopia, which is a centre for biodiversity of coffee species, but are widely grown in Africa and Latin America.

Coffee and tea were introduced to Europe and popularised between the late 16th and mid-17th century, as maritime trade grew around the world. Initially the drinks were promoted for their medicinal properties, but soon tea gardens and coffee houses sprang up all over Europe as people began to appreciate the pleasure tea and coffee gave. Although caffeine is the active ingredient, the flavours – which come from complex mixtures of volatile compounds in the tea and coffee plants – are an intrinsic part of the experience.

Latin America is also the source of another caffeine-containing drink, maté yerba which comes from leaves of the plant *Ilex paraguayensis*. In Africa, a drink is made from the caffeine-containing nuts of *Cola acuminata* and *Cola nitida*. The latter is, as the name suggests, the active ingredient of Coca-Cola, Pepsi-Cola and their brand imitation cola drinks. Coca-Cola was invented by Georgia pharmacist John Pemberton in 1886 and, yes, it did originally contain cocaine. But once the addictive properties of cocaine were realised in the early 20th century, it was removed from the drink and replaced with more caffeine.

There are other popular stimulants related chemically to caffeine. Theophylline and theobromine both occur in the cocoa plant from which chocolate is prepared. Theophylline is about as stimulating as caffeine, theobromine less so. Cocoa has long been used by people in the Amazon basin, Venezuela and Mexico as a drink called xocoatl. It was brought to the West by Christopher Columbus in 1492, and by Hernan Cortés, the conqueror of Mexico, in 1519.

Then there is guaranine, the active ingredient of guarana, a herbal stimulant made from the red berries of the plant *Paullinia cupana* which is native to the Amazon basin. Guarana drinks, tablets and powder are available from high-street chemists and health food shops. Plantations of *Paullinia cupana* for guarana production are being promoted in parts of Brazil by local co-operatives and environmental groups as a way of using rainforest sustainably.

Caffeine, and related stimulants, are white powders which are somewhat soluble in water, and also in organic solvents. The later property enables caffeine to be removed from coffee beans and tea leaves to make decaffeinated beverages. The beans or leaves are extracted with solvent in which the caffeine dissolves. Careful choice of solvent is necessary to ensure that not too many valuable flavour compounds are extracted along with the caffeine. The caffeine is then recovered from the solvent, and sold on to the drinks or pharmaceutical industry for addition to cola drinks or painkillers.

Caffeine and its relatives, belong to a group of compounds known as the xanthines, which are themselves part of a bigger group called the purines. All purines contain two fused rings of nitrogen and carbon atoms. Adenine and thymine are biologically important purines – they are important constituents of DNA. Adenine is also a component of adenosine triphosphate (ATP), the molecule which is a source of biochemical energy in all living things, and is often referred to as the energy 'currency' of the cell.

Coffee contains 100 milligrams of caffeine per average cup – about twice as much as a cup of tea. And a square of chocolate contains as much stimulant (caffeine, theophylline and theobromine) as a cup of tea. The average half-life of caffeine in the body is five to six hours – which explains why you may experience a sleepless night if you take coffee after dinner. Caffeine and related molecules are stripped down by liver enzymes to a basic xanthine nucleus, consisting of just the two fused rings, which is then excreted in the urine.

It has always been known that caffeine keeps you awake, but its mode of action was not appreciated until recently. It turns out that caffeine does not act like the other stimulants, cocaine and amphetamine. Instead of stimulating the brain directly, it inhibits the quietening of activity which occurs in neurons when we become sleepy. Adenosine, which is just adenine with a sugar molecule attached to it, appears to be one of the master molecules involved in sleep–wake cycles. All cellular activity is driven by ATP and as it gets used up, adenosine is produced as a waste product. Since there is, overall, more neuronal activity in the brain and the body when we are awake, more adenosine is produced during waking periods. But adenosine can also trigger a negative feedback loop, or brake, which damps down neuronal activity. Adenosine can dock onto specific adenosine receptors on neurons and inhibit their firing. In other words, as adenosine accumulates during the waking hours, it starts to quieten the brain and prepare the body for sleep by acting on these receptors.

There are two small patches of cells in the brain stem which are rich in adenosine receptors; these neurons contact all areas of the brain. So when the adenosine 'brake' is applied, the whole brain quietens down and we become sleepy. During the night, adenosine levels fall – because neurons are less active – so the receptors become unoccupied by adenosine molecules, releasing the brake and increasing alertness as neurons begin to fire again.

As we have seen, caffeine resembles adenosine in its molecular structure (the sugar group attached to the adenine is not important in this context) and it can block the action of adenosine by occupying its receptors. It cannot itself inhibit neuronal firing, so it acts as an antagonist rather than an agonist (see Chapter 1). With the adenosine brakes 'off' we stay awake. It may also enhance alertness by increasing levels of noradrenaline and adrenaline, although the mechanism for this is unknown.

But there appears to be more to caffeine than just increasing alertness. Artists, writers, and musicians throughout history have claimed that coffee, for instance, enhances creativity. Johann Sebastian Bach even wrote his famous Coffee Cantata in praise of his favourite drink. However, cognitive tests have so far failed to pin down exactly what effects caffeine has on mental performance. In general, caffeine drinks improve performance of simple tasks such as mental arithmetic or proof reading, but there is little evidence that it helps with more complex, demanding or creative activities. There is some suggestion that caffeine may boost neuronal firing, enhancing long-term potentiation and so improving memory.

As there are adenosine receptors elsewhere in the body, caffeine has a number of other physiological effects. It appears to boost physical endurance and can have a marked effect on athletic performance – so much so that caffeine is included, along with steroids, in the International Olympic Committee's list of restricted substances. The upper limit is 12 micrograms per millilitre of blood – the equivalent of six average cups of coffee in 30 minutes. Besides acting on adenosine receptors, caffeine may also release fat from cells for use as a fuel, which may help in running and jumping.

Caffeine also creates a small increase in the metabolic rate, probably by increasing adrenaline levels. Theoretically then, it could help in weight loss – particularly when coupled with the fat-release mechanism mentioned above; however, the effects are likely to be minimal.

One well-known side effect of caffeine is an increase in heart rate, and production of palpitations – again probably as a result of increased adrenaline. These symptoms often cause needless anxiety and disappear once caffeine consumption is decreased. Another noticeable side effect is an increase in the frequency of urination, which is caused by caffeine acting on adenosine receptors in the kidneys.

You may be surprised to learn that caffeine is a common ingredient of 'strong' painkillers (over-the-counter preparations that is, not prescription drugs such as morphine). There are two reasons for this. First, caffeine seems to enhance the effects of aspirin – by some as yet unknown mechanism. Second, adenosine acts on smooth muscle and plays a role in dilating blood vessels in the brain, which may lead to a so-called vascular headache (migraine is the commonest example of this kind of headache). By acting on adenosine receptors in these blood vessels, caffeine reverses this effect.

But sometimes caffeine use can actually *cause* vascular headaches. The blood vessels in the head may respond to long-term caffeine use by increasing their ability to dilate. Normally you do not notice this because regular intake of tea and coffee keeps the vessels contracted. Stop caffeine suddenly though, and the vessels will expand causing a so-called 'rebound' headache – to which the usual response is to go back to coffee or tea (or a caffeine-containing headache remedy) for relief. This interesting, and annoying, phenomenon was studied in a clinical context by doctors at the Hammersmith Hospital in London in 1989. They were able to uncover a clear link between post-operative headache – a very common experience after surgery – and the patient's previous level of caffeine consumption. In this situation, patients are forced to give up caffeine, temporarily, because no foods or beverages are allowed before an operation. Patients who drank four or more cups of tea a day were three times more likely to experience post-operative headache compared with those who drank one cup a day. A small number of patients in the study did not drink tea or coffee at all; none of these patients suffered a post-operative headache.

Other health effects of caffeine intake include a worsening of pre-menstrual syndrome in some women, because of complex interactions with female hormones. Some women find they can gain significant relief from the irritability, depression and fluid retention that hits them in the few days before their period by abstaining from tea and coffee at this time. Reports that caffeine – at moderate levels of consumption – is linked with pancreatic cancer, stomach cancer or heart disease have not been substantiated by further research. A study involving over 45,000 doctors whose caffeine intake and incidence of cardiovascular disease was monitored showed no link.

Cocaine and amphetamines are more powerful stimulants than caffeine and, unfortunately, are not nearly so benign. Cocaine, an extract from the coca plant *Erythroxylon coca*, which is cultivated the foothills of the Andes, has a very long history. It was extensively used in the Inca civilisation in Peru between the 10th and 15th centuries. Intially its use was restricted to priests and royalty for religious ceremonies and initiation rites. Later it spread to working people where it increased their stamina, enabling them to labour at high altitudes, while also taking their mind off hunger and other privations.

The Spanish conquerors of Peru in the 16th century encouraged the use of cocaine because it made their Indian subjects work so hard and kept them from complaining. But the drug did not enter European society in a big way until the 19th century. The German chemist Albert Niemann was the first to synthesise pure cocaine in 1860. It may seem incredible now, but there was even a tonic wine called Vin Mariani invented by the Sicilian Angelo Mariani which consisted of cocaine in wine. Touted as a cure for all ills, and endorsed by Pope Leo XIII, Vin Mariani was soon the most popular beverage in Europe, and was the forerunner to Coca-Cola (discussed above).

The father of psychoanalysis, Sigmund Freud, started to investigate cocaine for both scientific and personal reasons (he suffered from a number of ailments which had a nervous origin). In 1884 he published an influential essay 'Über Coca' which led to cocaine's widespread prescription for anxiety and depression – at least before its potential for addiction became known.

Amphetamines entered the drug culture in a quite different manner. In their chemical structure amphetamine resembles adrenaline. As we saw in

Chapter 4, noradrenaline is the 'flight or fight' hormone which is released by the adrenal glands in response to stress. One of the physiological effects of adrenaline is to expand the bronchi for faster, deeper breathing. It was thought, in the early 1900s, that adrenaline might be a good treatment for asthma, a condition characterised by contraction of the bronchi which leads to shortness of breath and wheezing. But adrenaline proved to be rather unstable if taken by mouth, so scientists at Eli Lilly (many years later to become the manufacturers of Prozac) began searching for an alternative. They found an old Chinese remedy in a shrub called ma huang or *Ephedra vulgaris*. The active ingredient was ephedrine (still used as a nasal decongestant). However, ma huang was scarce; in the course of synthesising ephedrine, chemists at Lilly came across a number of related compounds, including amphetamine. Later, they made metamphetamine, commonly known as 'speed'.

Amphetamine was first sold in inhaler form under the brand name Benzedrine. They were very widely available as an over-the-counter item in the 1930s and 1940s. Their use as an asthma remedy was forgotten, as people discovered the stimulating effects of ingesting the contents of a Benzedrine inhaler. Soon they were being used by students cramming for exams, tired housewives and, during World War II, by servicemen and civilians alike – on both sides of the conflict – to increase endurance and productivity. By this time amphetamine tablets were available. Amphetamines were sometimes prescribed for depression – at least before the anti-depressants were discovered, and sometimes even afterwards. A related compound methylphenidate (Ritalin) is widely used today, as discussed in the last chapter, for treatment of children with attention deficit disorder.

Amphetamines suppress appetite and were the first slimming drugs, although their official prescription for this purpose was stopped in the 1960s (they are still available in private slimming clinics today, although their use is heavily censured by the medical establishment).

Both cocaine and amphetamines produce a 'rush' of alertness, well-being and euphoria. Amphetamines closely resemble noradrenaline and, to a lesser extent, dopamine in their structure, but cocaine is less like either neurotransmitter. However, both drugs are sufficiently similar to enter into noradrenaline and dopamine-containing vesicles in neurons and displace the neurotransmitters, releasing them into the synapses. They also appear to inhibit their re-uptake.

The resultant enhanced levels of both noradrenaline and dopamine create a powerful stimulating effect. There is a high concentration of noradrenaline-containing neurons in the brain stem in an area called the locus coeruleus (meaning blue area, because the tissue here is literally blue). They spread out into both the limbic area and the cerebral cortex. Stimulation of the limbic area probably accounts for feelings of euphoria, while stimulation of the cortex will create alertness, energy, and clear thought. Injecting amphetamines, inhaling or 'snorting' cocaine or smoking 'crack' cocaine – a mixture of cocaine, baking powder, and water – cause a swift and intensely pleasurable response known as a 'rush' (the crack experience, in particular, has been called a 'whole body orgasm').

However, the 'rush' of a stimulant is generally followed by a 'crash' into depression. Worse, amphetamine use can produce a paranoid psychosis (which has, on occasion, led to the murder of the person thought to be plotting against the drug user). The symptoms resemble those of schizophrenia which, as we saw in the last chapter, is also associated with enhanced dopamine levels. Peculiar to amphetamine psychosis, though, are hallucinations of touch in which the user feels an intense itching or tingling, as if worms or small animals were crawling around under the skin.

The stimulant nicotine, which is the active ingredient of tobacco, has yet another mode of action. The origins of smoking are unknown, but Christopher Columbus saw Indians in Cuba smoking the leaves of the plant *Nicotiana tabacum*. Later, Sir Walter Raleigh noted natives of Virginia smoking leaves of a related species *Nicotiana rustica*. Both explorers played a part in introducing smoking into Europe, and the habit was widespread by the 17th century. Nicotine is a bitter, white substance, belonging to the chemical class called the alkaloids. These nitrogen-containing compounds have a wide range of structures, and occur in many different plants. They include many biologically active compounds such as morphine, strychnine and quinine (note, cocaine is also an alkaloid). It is named after the French ambassador to Portugal, Jean Nicot, who described it in 1560, although it was not isolated from the leaves until 1828.

When tobacco was first introduced into Europe, it was promoted as a panacea, perhaps because of its exotic origins. However, it was not long before people turned against it. King James I hated smoking and published a pamphlet against it. And smoking was banned in public in German-speaking Europe as early as 1649. However, governments were not blind to the fact that they could make money by taxing tobacco (so not much has changed).

Like many of the other alkaloids, nicotine is a poison in high enough doses. Sixty milligrams of nicotine placed on your tongue would kill you in minutes. A cigarette typically contains about one milligram of nicotine. It vapourises as the cigarette is smoked, forming minute droplets in the smoke which are rapidly absorbed into the bloodstream via the lungs, reaching the brain in about seven seconds.

Nicotine therefore has an almost immediate stimulating effect on the body. The neurotransmitter acetylcholine, which was discussed in the last chapter, has two kinds of receptor – known as nicotinic receptors and muscarinic receptors respectively. The former respond to nicotine, while the latter respond to muscarine, a toxin extracted from the fly agaric mushroom *Amanita muscaria*. The physiological effects of nicotine therefore resemble those of acetylcholine in both the brain and the autonomic nervous system. Blood pressure increases (making smoking a risk factor for heart disease), heart rate increases, and pupils dilate. The effects of stimulating nicotinic receptors in the brain are decreased appetite and – perhaps – enhanced memory and concentration. This is also presumably the source of the pleasure of smoking – although the exact mechanism involved is not fully understood.

Smoking kills because of the carcinogenic tars created when tobacco burns. When these are inhaled, they set the scene for cancer – especially lung cancer. Nicotine itself is not so directly harmful. It kills because it is addictive, which leads smokers to carry on smoking, continuing their exposure to tars.

Alcohol – simple molecule, complex drug

Alcohol – or ethanol, to give it the correct chemical name – is the world's most popular recreational drug, after caffeine. Recent analysis of stains inside an Iranian pottery jar suggests that wine-making dates back to the Neolithic era (5400–5000 BC). The ancient Greeks and Romans drank wine, while beer was made in medieval monasteries. Alcohol differs from the other recreational drugs we have looked at so far in that it has to be created – rather than extracted. The details of how yeast turns sugar into alcohol were not worked out until 1939.

Ethanol also differs from most other drugs in being a rather small molecule – consisting of just two carbon atoms, six hydrogen atoms and one oxygen atom. A standard drink or unit of an alcoholic drink (a glass of wine or half a pint of beer) contains about 8 grams of alcohol. Once inside the body it is mostly absorbed by the small intestine and then proceeds to the liver and from there to the rest of the body – as do all other drugs. However, many of the molecules may be broken down by an enzyme called alcohol dehydrogenase (ADH) in either the stomach or in the liver. ADH can deal with about one unit of alcohol an hour. Drink faster than this, and the level of alcohol in the blood will steadily increase. Women have less ADH activity than men, which is why they usually show both the short and long-term effects of alcohol more readily, and on a smaller intake.

The actions of alcohol are quite complex. It acts as a general depressant in the nervous system by interfering with glutamate receptors; this has an inhibitory effect on the corresponding neuron. This results in a number of different effects. In the region of the cerebral cortex, neural circuits concerning judgement and discretion may be inhibited resulting in talkative, reckless behaviour and maybe even aggression. Neurons in the area to do with balance and speech may also be inhibited, resulting in unco-ordinated movement, and slurred speech – at least at higher alcohol intakes. At very high intakes neurons controlling heart rate and breathing may be affected, possibly leading to death (a bottle of whisky consumed at one sitting has been known to be fatal). And of course glutamate is involved in long-term potentiation and memory. Memories formed when not drinking are not wiped out, but new memories are not so easily formed under the influence of alcohol – leading to the familiar hangover symptom of not being able to remember what happened at a party where much alcohol was consumed (however, the extremes of an alcoholic blackout seem to result from more than glutamate receptor inhibition).

But alcohol has other effects in the brain. Like Valium, it binds to GABA receptors (as discussed in the last chapter), although not on the same site as the tranquilliser. This produces a welcome antidote to stress – but also makes alcohol especially dangerous when used in conjunction with tranquillisers, as it will potentiate their effect, which could be fatal. And alcohol can also increase dopamine levels in the limbic system – although it is not known quite how this happens. This gives rise to pleasurable feelings which resemble the 'rush' described above for cocaine and amphetamines, although they are not as intense. And finally, alcohol can act rather like morphine, because it can release endorphins from the pituitary gland. However, since alcohol does not act directly on endorphin receptors the sensation will be weaker than the morphine experience.

Alcohol acts as a depressant in sexual function. By acting on glutamate receptors in the peripheral nervous system, it can inhibit the blood vessels in the penis, vagina and clitoris from dilating in response to sexual stimuli. Thus, the sex organs cannot engorge with blood, which is a prerequisite to physiological sexual arousal. However, in psychological experiments people taking alcohol often report *feeling* more aroused; the problem is that drinking inhibits the physical means to carry out their desires.

Drinking a moderate amount also seems to confer some immunity from infection. In a recent study, regular wine drinkers reported fewer colds and bouts of flu. In test-tube experiments, red wine showed a remarkable ability to kill microbes – so maybe alcohol has an antibiotic effect. However, too much alcohol is also known to undermine the immune system. And of course, moderate drinking appears to cut the risk of cardiovascular disease – as was discussed in Chapter 5. A recent study by French scientists showed another health benefit – moderate wine consumption (three to four glasses a day) appears to protect against the development of dementia in the over-65s.

However, there is little doubt that alcohol can be a very dangerous drug when taken in excess. The problem of alcohol addiction will be discussed below. People who drink in binges run the risk of being involved in accidents or violent crime and are more likely to commit suicide. And even if you stop short of a binge, you will be in no doubt of alcohol's toxic effects when you suffer a hangover.

Alcohol acts as a diuretic, increasing urination, because it inhibits the production of vasopressin from the pituitary gland. Vasopressin usually acts on the kidneys, controlling the amount of water they excrete from the body. The net effect is that if you drink a glass of wine, you lose twice that volume from your body as urine. Unless this is made up by drinking more water, a dry mouth and bad breath will result from dehydration – which is also a potent factor in causing a headache.

However, it is not alcohol itself but acetaldehyde, the breakdown product from the action of ADH, which produces most of the unpleasant symptoms of a hangover. Acetaldehyde produces nausea and headache. These pass with time, as the next enzyme in line – acetaldehyde dehydrogenase – turns acetaldehyde into harmless acetic acid. Then there are congeners, the chemicals found in dark drinks like red wine, brandy and rum, which may also be potent toxins. Add to this the fact that alcohol interferes with normal sleep cycles, producing fatigue the following day, and it is easy to see why there is no perfect cure for a hangover; it is just physiologically too complex an event.

Expanding the mind – the experience of psychedelic drugs

Perhaps the most awesome (some would say alarming) of the recreational drugs are those which can create profound changes in perception and self-awareness – sometimes resulting in mystical or religious experiences. These are the psychedelic drugs. Although some people still call them hallucinogens, this is not a very accurate description of their effects. A true hallucination is a perception occurring in the absence of an environmental stimulus. In the psychedelic experience, you are more likely to experience distortion of perceptions – the colour of a leaf or flower will seem exceptionally intense, or an object in the room will suddenly acquire immense significance, for example. Extraordinary images and patterns are commonly seen behind closed eyes, and the sense of time and space is often altered, with an hour seeming like a year and the length of a room like a hundred miles. A common, and awe-inspiring, experience on psychedelic drugs is an expanded sense of the self, as if the boundaries between the ego and the rest of the world had dissolved.

The psychedelic experience varies in intensity from the gentle relaxation produced by smoking cannabis, to the full-blown 'trip' induced by LSD or mescaline. Psychedelics are a quite diverse group of compounds. Some, like psilocybin and mescaline, are derived from natural products (mushrooms and the peyote cactus), while others – Ecstasy and LSD – are the product of the chemistry laboratory.

The role played by psychedelic drugs in human culture has changed over their long history. Magic mushrooms and peyote have been used in religious rituals in Mexico and Central America for hundreds of years. In the 19th and early 20th centuries the chemists got their hands on these substances and began to extract and identify their active ingredients.

Some prominent figures have been remarkably frank in describing their experiences on psychedelic drugs. British writer Aldous Huxley wrote of his 12 hour mescaline 'trip' in *The Doors of Perception*. And Swiss chemist Albert Hofmann got more than he bargained for when he discovered LSD; he appears to have ingested some of the compound and was overcome by a dizziness and restlessness which forced him to abandon his day's work in the laboratory. When he lay down, eyes closed, at home he was overcome by the LSD experience – strange shapes, bizarre visions, and a fantastic interplay of colours. He, and colleagues, went on to study the effects of LSD by dosing themselves deliberately and recording the effects.

Between the 1950s and 1970s some psychiatrists and psychotherapists researched the potential of psychedelic drugs for the treatment of mental illnesses and less severe psychological problems. For instance, LSD was used by Stanislav Grof as a way of gaining a better understanding of schizophrenia. Grof's experiments, carried out in Czechoslovakia and the United

States, are described in his book *Realms of the Human Unconscious*. Ecstasy was used in marital therapy as an aid to facilitate the breakdown of barriers between couples by creating feelings of empathy.

But most of this research was stopped, because of concern over the increasing use of psychedelics in the general population in the 1960s. LSD, in particular, was at the heart of the cultural revolution that swept young people worldwide at this time. Use of the drug was promoted by figures such as Timothy Leary in the United States, while figures in the pop world, such as the Beatles, made allusions to psychedelic experiences in their songs.

Today psychedelics are as popular as ever, but the emphasis has changed. In the 1960s people were more interested in exploring their inner worlds with LSD. From the late 1980s, the drugs – and Ecstasy in particular – have been used more for pure enjoyment and creating friendly feelings within a group of people. Ecstasy is part and parcel of the clubbing and dance culture of the West, and pop lyrics now reflect this rather than the bizarre symbols of the LSD experience.

The four most widely used psychedelics are cannabis, Ecstasy, LSD and magic mushrooms. Like so many of the drugs discussed here, cannabis has a long history. It was widely used for medicinal purposes in Europe and the United States in the 19th century – and even had the seal of royal approval, for Queen Victoria was prescribed it for relief of menstrual cramps. Cannabis, sometimes also known as hemp, comes from the plant *Cannabis sativa*, which is widely cultivated in the Middle East, Asia and North Africa (and even in Britain). It is consumed in two main forms. The dried flowering tops of the plant are smoked in a form called marijuana, while the resin from the plant, which can be smoked or eaten in cakes or biscuits, is known as hashish.

Cannabis takes effect very quickly; it is both relaxing and alters perception, particularly of space and time (without being overtly hallucinogenic). Higher doses may produce some adverse effects, such as anxiety, panic and paranoia. Cannabis contains many closely related active compounds called cannabinoids, of which the most important is tetrahydrocannabinol (THC). This was identified in 1964 by the Israeli chemist Raphael Mechoulam. More recently, it has been shown that neurons contain a specific cannabinoid receptor. This invites comparison with the opiate drugs, such as heroin, which also have specific receptors. Mechoulam kept his scientific interest in cannabis going and, in 1993, announced the discovery of the natural ligand for the cannabinoid receptor, a molecule called anandamide (from the Sanskrit word ananda, meaning bliss).

This opens the way to the development of drugs based on THC – not for relaxation and enjoyment, but for medical purposes. It has long been known that cannabis has a number of therapeutic effects. For instance, it can relieve the pressure of the fluid inside the eyeball in glaucoma. Left unchecked this fluid presses on the optic nerve and threatens the eyesight. Cannabis also relieves muscle spasticity, urinary incontinence and pain in multiple sclerosis, it alleviates the nausea that accompanies cancer chemotherapy and stimulates appetite in AIDS. For these reasons, many thousands of patients use cannabis illegally (sometimes tacitly encouraged by their doctors). Consequently, there is a strong campaign to legalise the medical use of cannabis and to promote further research into its applications.

Currently, pharmaceutical companies steer clear of such research because of the 'shady' associations of cannabis and, of course, because it cannot be patented as a new drug. There is currently just one synthetic cannabinoid drug on the market, nabilone, used as an oral treatment for nausea produced by cancer chemotherapy. Nabilone does not seem to have any psychoactive effects.

If legal restrictions were lifted there could be other advantages; cannabis is easily cultivated, and therefore cheap. The cannabis plant has other uses: its fibres can be used to make paper, textiles, or rope – indeed it was widely used in this way in the 19th century and is now cultivated again for these purposes in Britain (but the crop contains little THC). And were its recreational use sanctioned, it could compete with cigarettes, tranquillisers, and alcohol as a stress-reliever. No wonder that supporters of the medical use of cannabis hint darkly at vested interests in the tobacco and drinks industry as the driving forces against legalisation.

In contrast to cannabis, Ecstasy has a purely hedonistic image. Its chemical name is 3,4-methylenedioxymetamphetamine or MDMA for short. It goes by an ever-changing variety of pseudonyms such as 'Adam' (there is a closely related drug called 'Eve'), Love Dove, Rhubarb and Custard and so on. As the name suggests, MDMA is an amphetamine, but also has psychedelic qualities. There are hundreds of similar compounds – some purely synthetic, others derived from natural substances such as nutmeg and crocuses. Over the years, researchers tried to find a therapeutic use for MDMA, but failed. It resurfaced as a recreational drug in the 1980s (a related drug, MDA entered popular culture earlier, in the 1960s and was nicknamed 'The Love Drug'). It comes from illicit laboratories – many of them in the Netherlands – and is sold in tablet form, often adulterated with other substances, which may or may not have some psychoactive effect.

As an amphetamine derivative, Ecstasy increases dopamine levels and so gives a powerful energy rush, which enables users to party all night. But there is another dimension; it creates euphoria, loving feelings towards others, and enhances perceptions. This is thought to be due, in part at least, to some serotonin-boosting effect which the drug has. A tablet contains 75–100 milligrams of Ecstasy, and the effects kick in after 20 to 60 minutes, lasting for several hours. Physiological effects include dilation of the pupils, sweating, dry mouth, and increase in heart rate, blood pressure and body temperature.

Weekend use of Ecstasy is common, with abstinence between times. Although deaths after taking Ecstasy have received much publicity, particularly in the UK, they are still rare. However, the combination of high blood pressure and increased body temperature is potentially very dangerous as heat stroke may occur, especially in people who keep on dancing when they are already very hot. Attempting to cool off by then downing gallons of water can be catastrophic, for this is one of the few occasions when water can actually be toxic. What happens is that the blood gets diluted in the sense that its salt concentration decreases. The brain absorbs this excess fluid like a sponge, swells enormously and is crushed by the skull. To rehydrate on Ecstasy it is best to use the same regime which is recommended for severe diarrhoea – take water, but add a teaspoon of salt per litre, or better still use specially formulated 'isotonic' sports drinks. Most deaths though, occur from widespread blood clotting which can occur under conditions of heat stroke, or from heart failure.

Some people report a depressive crash after Ecstasy use, and there have also been reports of occasional liver damage from use of the drug. Lack of research into Ecstasy accounts for the shortage of data on its long-term effects. For this we will have to rely on ancedotal reports in the future from the millions of young people, on either side of the Atlantic, who take Ecstasy on a regular basis.

The psychoactive effects of cannabis and Ecstasy pale into insignificance when compared to the experience of a full-blown LSD trip. Lysergic acid diethylamide, as has been mentioned, was synthesised by Hofmann in 1943. He had been investigating the compounds of ergot, an extract from the fungus *Claviceps purpura* which is a parasite of rye wheat. Since the Middle Ages it has been known that ergot has both medicinal and toxic properties. It was used to contract the uterus and so hasten childbirth; the active ingredient was found to be the compound ergonovine. Another compound, ergotamine, contracts blood vessels in the scalp and is used today as a migraine treatment. The common structure for all the ingredients of ergot is lysergic acid, discovered by chemists at New York's Rockefeller Institute. Hofmann was working for the Sandoz company on synthetic derivatives of lysergic acid, when he made LSD. Incidentally, hydergine – the 'smart' drug which was discussed in the last chapter – emerged from the same research programme. As with Ecstasy, no therapeutic uses for LSD have been established. Further, no definite mechanism has yet been established for its spectacular effects – although it has been assumed that the drug may act on the serotonin system, because the LSD molecule partly resembles serotonin.

Nowadays, LSD is used in smaller doses than in the heady days of the 1960s – 50 micrograms per 'tab' rather than 250. Use of LSD gives rise to few adverse physical effects, but can on occasion – and even after a single use – trigger a schizophrenia-like illness. And the sometimes tragic effects of a bad 'trip' are well known, with users acting on some of their drug-induced illusions – leaping out of high windows, believing they could fly, for instance. Another problem is troubling 'flashbacks' of the LSD experience which may occur weeks or even months after the drug is taken.

Albert Hofmann was also involved in the discovery of the active ingredients of magic mushrooms. It is impossible to check compounds for psychedelic effects on animals, so Hofmann had to try out the extracts on himself. He noted that two compounds, psilocybin and psilocin, had an effect very similar to LSD – hardly surprising since they too resemble serotonin. Dedicated drug users who want a cheap high pick magic mushrooms during the fruiting season from September to November. The best species is the Liberty Cap, which contains psilocybin.

There is no simple explanation in terms of neurotransmitters for the remarkable effects of psychedelic drugs. Although all the compounds we have discussed resemble serotonin, noradrenaline and dopamine, experiments have shown that they do not act on receptors in a predictable way. Work done by George Aghajanian at Yale University has focused attention on the locus coeruleus, which contains a high concentration of noradrenaline neurons. Sensory stimuli cause these neurons to fire at an accelerated rate and psychedelic drugs cause them to fire even more. This may produce a hyper-responsiveness to external stimuli – sounds, sights and touch – which could create enhanced perception. In particular, accelerated activity in the locus coeruleus may explain synaesthesia, a phenomenon in which perceptions are 'mixed'. Notes are 'seen' in the mind's eye as colours, while touch can be experienced as sound. Synaesthesia is common under the influence of LSD. If all stimuli are funnelled through the locus coeruleus it is possible that the signals could become mixed once processed higher up in the brain, and mixing could be more likely if the locus is more stimulated. And as we have already noted, the locus coeruleus contacts nearly all part of the brain. Enhanced stimulation could create a condition of enhanced awareness which may be experienced as an expanded sense of self.

The other face of opiates

We have met the opiate drugs in Chapter 6, where their action as painkillers was discussed. They have been widely used for both medicinal and recreational purposes since the 16th century, particularly in the form of laudanum (the name coming from the Latin laudare, which means to praise) which was a tincture of opium. Opium was used by writers such as Edgar Allen Poe, Thomas de Quincey and Samuel Coleridge. The influence of opium is obvious in some of the lines of Coleridge's *Rime of the Ancient Mariner*, while de Quincey became famous after the publication of his drug-taking memoir *Confessions of an English Opium Eater* in 1821.

Nowadays, the opiate most often taken for recreational use is heroin – a synthetic derivative of morphine (and strictly speaking therefore called an opioid). Heroin can still be prescribed for relief of severe pain in, for example, terminal cancer although its recreational use is generally associated with severe penalties.

Heroin, a white powder, can be sniffed, smoked or injected. Heating the powder and inhaling the fumes through a small tube is a popular means of administration known as 'chasing the dragon'. The drug takes effect very quickly. It appears to alter the perception of psychological as well as physical pain; it has a generally cushioning effect often described as like being wrapped in cotton wool. Like morphine it acts on opiate receptors, mimicking the action of the body's natural 'feel good' chemicals, the endorphins, only in a more intense way. Heroin is notorious because, as with many of the other drugs we have considered here, it produces dependence – which will be discussed below.

A survey of recreational drug use

Consumption of caffeine around the world is nearly universal, in some form. Alcohol is the next most popular recreational drug. Ninety per cent of people in the UK drink it, and similar figures apply to the rest of the

Western world. However, alcohol is banned in some Middle Eastern states for religious reasons. Tobacco comes next; while smoking is decreasing in the West, 28 per cent of UK men and 26 per cent of women still smoke, and the figures are even higher for school-age children. Seventy-two per cent of girls aged 15 to 16 smoke, and 63 per cent of boys. In the 11–15 age group 13 per cent of girls and 12 per cent of boys are regular smokers. And smoking is on the increase in developing countries, such as China, as the tobacco industry increasingly targets its marketing efforts in these regions. Smoking and drinking are both higher in Eastern Europe than in the West.

When it comes to so-called illicit drug use data is less reliable as few large surveys have been carried out. However, some interesting observations can be discerned from the figures that are available. Cannabis is, by far, the most popular drug – with 2.5 per cent of the world's population using it. Heroin is the least used drug, with only 0.14 per cent of people admitting to its consumption. Usage is, however, higher than this in Asia, Europe and Oceania and lower in the Americas. LSD, cocaine and amphetamines come somewhere in between.

In Britain, one person in four says they have used illicit drugs at one time, with usage being concentrated in the under-35 age group, and five per cent are using the drugs currently. Eighty per cent of these use cannabis. Around one in ten has used amphetamines, LSD, magic mushrooms or Ecstasy – which is hardly surprising given the popularity of the dance and clubbing culture in Europe. Only 1–2 per cent of the general population use heroin or cocaine, and fewer than 1 per cent say they have ever injected a drug. This pattern is not dissimilar to the rest of Europe, although drug consumption is relatively high in the UK, as it also appears to be in some Mediterranean countries – maybe because they are close to supply routes. Another difference is that there is much more poly-drug use in the UK than elsewhere – that is, people use more than one drug at a time, or will switch from one drug to another if their drug of choice is not available.

But why do so many people take recreational drugs? At first the answer seems obvious – they give pleasure, as has been described in the preceding section. However, there must be much more to it than this. Many people abstain from drugs entirely, while others become dependent (of which more later) and take them even when the problems they cause far outweigh the pleasure they give.

There are a number of explanations for this individual variation in drug-taking behaviour. Like diabetics who lack insulin, some people may be naturally deficient in brain chemicals such as endorphins or serotonin and unconsciously self-medicate with recreational drugs. For young people, peer-group pressure, sensation-seeking, curiosity, and adolescent rebellion probably play a major role in drug taking. In the UK, two children out of five have tried an illicit drug by the time they take their GCSEs (at 15–16), with one in ten having taken Ecstasy or LSD. And at all ages, some people just prefer the instant gratification that can be obtained from drug taking to delayed satisfactions, such as a house, car or holiday in the sun paid for from careful saving.

Most people are well able to control their drug intake, whatever their motivation for using them. However, many recreational drugs have the potential for creating dependence – and in this situation users expose themselves to a wide range of physical, psychological and social problems.

Dependence (also known as addiction) is a complex phenomenon resulting from an interaction between the drug, the individual user and the environment. The road to dependence usually starts with tolerance, which is the need to take increasing amounts of the drug to create the same effect. The molecular mechanisms of tolerance are not completely understood, but are related to the way in which the body responds to repeated administration of a drug. Liver enzymes may increase their activity, degrading the drug more rapidly so that the effective concentration in the body is decreased – creating the need for an increased dosage. Or the brain may respond to the effects of the drug, be it stimulating or sedating, by attempting to restore the status quo (just another of the many homeostatic mechanisms which allows the body to function in a stable way).

Tolerance leads to withdrawal symptoms. When the drug is withdrawn, the brain and body may respond with a range of symptoms which are usually the opposite to those created by the drug; so the sedating effects of heavy alcohol use could lead to withdrawal effects of shaking and even convulsions. The origin of withdrawal symptoms is probably the same as that of tolerance – the brain and body compensate for the presence of the drug by trying to neutralise its effect. All the time the drug is being taken, this compensation is masked – although it requires increasing doses to achieve this. Remove the drug and the compensation mechanism reveals itself as withdrawal symptoms.

Both tolerance and withdrawal symptoms may promote increased usage of the drug. Tolerance means the user needs more to get the desired effect, while withdrawal means they need more to block the unpleasant symptoms. But greater usage in itself creates more tolerance and withdrawal, as the brain fights harder to correct the imbalances induced by the drug.

Increasingly the user is drawn into a vicious circle. Dependence is a subtle mix of physical and psychological components – the latter related to the user being compelled to function according to the brain's altered chemistry. The result is an obsession with the drug, and the user's life starts to revolve around drug-seeking behaviour.

Some drugs are more likely to produce dependence than others. This list bears no relation to their legality. Alcohol, nicotine, cocaine and – most of all – heroin are definitely addictive. There is even some evidence that caffeine may be mildly addictive in a minority of users.

More people are addicted to nicotine than to any other drug. Most people who try to give up fail repeatedly. Yet one in two smokers will die from the habit – not from nicotine, but from the tars in cigarette, cigar and pipe smoke.

Alcohol dependence is the second most common addiction. Doctors make a distinction between people who are alcohol dependent (formerly known as alcoholics) and problem drinkers. The former have the full-blown syndrome of tolerance and withdrawal symptoms – which include tremor, agitation, and even fits. The problem drinker, who may drink in binges and has alcohol-related problems such as drink-driving and aggression, is harder to spot. Alcohol misuse is usually diagnosed by psychological questionnaire coupled with blood and urine tests. The scale of the problem is huge with perhaps 9 per cent of men and 5 per cent of women having alcohol problems. A recent survey showed that the number of women drinking more than the (then) recommended limit of 14 units per week has increased to 14 per cent in the UK – with the increase being concentrated in professional, high-income women who drink to relieve stress, and to keep up with their professional male counterparts. (Since the survey was carried out, the UK minimum recommended alcohol limit for women has been raised to 21 units a week, and 28 for men). There is also a large increase in the number of over-65s of both sexes drinking more than is recommended.

Problem drinkers have two to three times the mortality risk of the general population from accidents, suicide, liver damage and other health problems. They also take twice as much time off work and run the risk of brain damage and several types of cancer, to say nothing of the social cost in terms of damaged relationships with friends and family.

As far as other dependencies are concerned, the figures rely – in the UK at least – on notifications to the Home Office of people with opiate or cocaine addiction by the doctors treating them. In 1995, the last year for which figures are available, the number was 37,164 – two-thirds of whom were heroin-dependent. This probably represents about one in five of people with a heroin problem. Heroin users run a 20 to 30 times greater risk of mortality than the rest of the population. One per cent of them die from overdose, suicide or drug-related disease. If HIV infection from needle sharing is taken into account, then this figure rises to 4 per cent.

There are many possible causes for drug dependence of all kinds. There is a genetic factor; children of alcoholics have four times the risk of the general population of becoming dependent on alcohol themselves. Ken Blum of the University of Texas claims to have found a gene that could be responsible for alcohol and other dependencies. This codes for a defective dopamine receptor. If the reward/pleasure system described above is defective, then drug-seeking behaviour to remedy this would not be surprising. And there are recent reports from the University of Oregon of alcohol-dependent mice who have a defect in a serotonin receptor. This would fit in nicely with observations that alcoholics do tend to have low serotonin activity, and alcohol increases it (remember, from the last chapter, that Prozac tends to decrease alcohol consumption).

Environmental factors are important in drug dependence. A study of US soldiers in the Vietnam War who had become dependent on heroin showed that most remained 'clean' once they returned home. And studies with other drug-dependent people show they experience cravings when they are exposed to cues such as drug preparation. The importance of environmental cues has also been demonstrated in animal models.

The search for the addictive personality has been, so far, unfruitful. The most thorough personality questionnaire – the Minnesota Multiphasic Personality Inventory – was administered to students of the University of Minnesota between 1947 and 1961. Later, links between personality and drug dependence were investigated and came up with no positive results, strongly suggesting that dependent drug users have normal personalities.

Inevitably, there have been many studies of drug dependence using brain scans. The problem with such techniques, which study the biochemistry of the brain, is that you cannot be sure that abnormalities are not actually produced by the usage of the drug, rather than being a predisposing factor.

Ultimately, it should be possible to explain drug dependence in molecular terms, using techniques and theories similar to those described in the last chapter. Drugs of dependence are all very dissimilar in their chemical structures and mode of action, so what is the common factor which leads to dependence?

It is possible to study drug dependence in an animal model, as Barry

Everitt of Cambridge University and others have shown. Rats can be allowed to press a lever for delivery of a potentially addictive drug. It has been shown that the animals will press the lever thousands of times, ignoring food and water, for a drug like cocaine. Other experiments have suggested that the drugs of dependence work on the brain's reward centre, which is located in a small region of the mid brain called the nucleus accumbens. There are dopamine-driven connections between this area and both the cerebral cortex and the limbic system which are thought to have an evolutionary value in creating pleasure after eating or sex. Drugs that enhance these pathways at various points short-circuit the route to pleasure and may account for the psychological aspect of dependence. Further research suggests repeated application of these drugs may actually cause permanent changes in the neural circuits in this region which account for the characteristics of dependence. It appears that the memory protein, CREB, which was discussed in the last chapter, may be involved in this remodelling process. Mice deficient in CREB show milder withdrawal symptoms from opiates than normal mice.

Treatments for drug dependence

All people dependent on drugs – from nicotine to heroin – benefit from psychological treatments which tackle the roots of their behaviour. Beyond this, however, there are some drug treatments which may be helpful.

People trying to give up smoking can treat themselves with decreasing amounts of nicotine (gradual withdrawal of addictive drugs gives the body time to adjust to abstinence). Nicotine patches and chewing gum are helpful – although it is regrettable that there is not more help for people caught up in this most common form of drug addiction.

There are pharmaceutical therapies too for people with alcohol problems. The most well-established – and controversial – is disulfiram or Antabuse, which induces the production of acetaldehyde, resulting in a concentrated hangover. Intense nausea deters the user from consuming alcohol. Antabuse is available as a challenging six month implant, or as a daily tablet (which of course an alcoholic can stop taking at any time).

Two more benign drugs have been used to treat alcohol problems in recent years. Naltrexone, which is an antagonist at opiate receptors and also used to treat opiate addiction, reduces the pleasure of drinking. The mechanism is not well understood, but it could be that the opiate receptor system interacts in some way with the reward system.

More recently, acamprosate has been used for alcohol dependence. This mimics the effects of alcohol by both boosting the effects of GABA and blocking NMDA – but without creating dependence. In a practical sense it relieves the craving for a drink. In clinical trials, after one year of treatment with either acamprosate or placebo and with follow-up of one year, 39 per cent remained abstinent in the treatment group, compared with 17 per cent who received placebo.

The standard treatment for opiate addiction is methadone. This is an opioid given in tablet form which does not give the same high as heroin, although it is still addictive. The aim of methadone treatment is harm reduction – weaning the addict away from a drug-dependent lifestyle and minimising the dangers of injecting and environmental cues. More recently other drugs such as buprenorphine and LAAM have been used as methadone analogues.

The above drugs provide a long-term solution to drug dependence. However, there are also some 'quick fixes'. Drug withdrawal under anaesthetic has been tried recently with good results. So too has a drug called ibogaine, isolated from the West African shrub *Tabernanthe iboga*. This has been pioneered by the former US addict Howard Lotsof, who has worked with patients in the Netherlands and claims a 75 per cent success rate. On adminstration of ibogaine, patients enter a waking dream, in which their life flashes before them and they are able to reflect on and solve any problems which may have lead to drug-taking behaviour. In animal experiments, ibogaine stops drug-seeking behaviour.

And in the most recent development, it may be possible to immunise vulnerable people against drug dependence. Most of the research has been done with cocaine, for which there is currently no drug therapy. Antibodies to cocaine break down the drug in the body before it reaches the brain, which should stop the development of dependence. Tests in humans begin in 1998.

Humans always have, and always will, indulge in recreational drugs – for relaxation, pleasure and inspiration. The challenge is to learn more about how they act on the brain, so that dependence and the accompanying physical and mental harm can be avoided.

With recreational drugs, people take the use of biologically active compounds into their own hands, without the sanction of the medical 'authorities'. And there is another type of 'do it yourself' in drug consumption. In the next chapter we look at how people are turning increasingly to the alternative pharmacy represented by the health food shop, and using vitamins, minerals and herbs alongside – or instead of – pharmaceutical drugs.

10

Natural alternatives: vitamins, minerals and herbs

As we saw in the last chapter, people can choose to take drugs for non-medical reasons. Here we review the way people take non-drugs for medical reasons. These non-drugs are mostly classified – at least in the UK – as food supplements. Unlike the pharmaceutical drugs discussed in other chapters, these are mostly substances found naturally in the human diet, such as vitamins and minerals. Herbal extracts are also increasingly popular, and although many of these would not normally find their way into the average Western diet, they are still classified as food supplements.

The reason for this classification is to avoid taking the products through the development and testing processes described in Chapter 2. Often this is a reasonable choice; most of these products have been in use for hundreds of years, so clinical testing can be regarded as having been done – albeit in an informal way. So if vitamin C, one of the most popular supplements, were in any way seriously toxic we should have heard about it by now.

Pharmaceutical companies, on the whole, are unlikely to take on the licensing of any vitamin, herb or related product. Their long tradition of use means that they cannot be patented and therefore companies will not be able to gain back finance invested in development from royalties. This leaves manufacturers of these 'natural' medicines free to promote their products, although they may not advertise these as if they were licensed drugs. Compare the detailed description of a prescription medicine with the vague wording on a packet of vitamin C or evening primrose oil to see the difference several million pounds of research and development makes.

It could be argued that those who sell food supplements have it both ways. Walking into a health food shop, or even a high street chemist, gives the strong impression that an 'alternative' form of pharmacy has sprung up. If supplements fail to deliver, or if they actually harm you, then the manufacturer bears little responsibility.

The supplements industry is growing year on year. Partly this is due to increasing disillusionment with the pharmaceutical industry and the search for medicines that serve unmet needs, and partly to the wish of an ageing population to keep itself in good health. In the UK, we spend more on supplements than we do on over-the-counter analgesics. In 1996, we spent £296 million on supplements, compared to £185 million on painkillers. Thirty-nine per cent of the population spends on supplements, with the highest spenders being in the over-50s age group. The market is predicted to grow dramatically into the 21st century. Cod liver oil is the most popular supplement, followed by multivitamins, iron, vitamin C and garlic. In the US, around $5 billion a year is spent on vitamins and minerals, and the market is said to be growing by 20 per cent annually. Yet all these substances are available in the human diet. The money spent on supplements could be used to stock up on vitamin and mineral-rich foods. So is there any scientific rationale for taking them at all?

Vitamins and minerals: the case for supplementation

The main constituents of our daily diet are carbohydrates, fats and proteins. These fuel the body and provide the raw ingredients for building vital molecules such as enzymes, hormones, and DNA. Vitamins and minerals are important constituents of enzymes and carry out a number of other roles – for instance, sodium and potassium are vital for the transmission of nerve impulses. It has long been known that deficiencies of specific vitamins and minerals can lead to disease. For instance, sailors on long voyages in the 16th and 17th centuries would commonly suffer scurvy – characterised by anaemia and repeated infection – due to lack of vitamin C. This was remedied by Scots physician James Lind in around 1750 by the supply of adequate amounts of citrus fruits to sailors on board ship. However, vitamin C and the other vitamins were not isolated and identified until the 20th century. Similarly the role of minerals was not appreciated until the science of modern biochemistry was developed.

Knowledge of the importance of vitamins and minerals led nutritional experts to formulate recommended daily allowances (RDAs) for these so-called micronutrients. For instance, the current RDA for vitamin C is 60 mg, while that for zinc is 15 mg. The RDAs however, vary with the age and sex of the individual and with their circumstances; smokers are said to need more vitamin C, for instance. Some nutrition experts think the RDAs are too low and do not take account of the vitamin and mineral content of the modern diet, or of current health issues. Andrew Weil, qualified medic and complementary health specialist, (voted one of America's most influential men by *Time* magazine) recommends taking up to 6 *grams* a day of vitamin C. A similar prescription was put forward many years previously by double Nobel Prize winner, the chemist Linus Pauling. People, on the whole, dismissed Pauling as a crank. The signs are that Weil is taken more seriously.

If vitamins and minerals do have a role to play in modern times, when obvious deficiency diseases are rare, then it is as antioxidants which can protect from degenerative diseases such as cancer, arthritis, cataract and, as discussed briefly in Chapter 5, cardiovascular disease. Antioxidants ward off the cellular ageing processes that set the scene for these diseases.

One of the quirks of evolution is our need for oxygen, a naturally occurring chemical which is ultimately toxic to us. When life first emerged on earth in the form of blue–green algae, sometimes also known as cyanobacteria, nearly four billion years ago, it did not need oxygen to survive. These bacteria probably lived in a global atmosphere dominated by the gas carbon dioxide. It was only as evolution progressed that more complex organisms, which used oxygen to dismantle food molecules to extract energy, began to dominate. The anaerobes, which lived without oxygen (it was toxic to some, others tolerated it) retreated. Today the ancestors of these ancient organisms are found in low-oxygen environments, such as compost heaps, the ocean floor, stagnant ponds, and the human gut.

Oxygen is toxic mainly because it is the second most reactive element on earth (the most reactive is fluorine which, unlike oxygen, does not occur naturally in its elemental state – so we need not worry about it). When oxygen reacts with glucose – which it does very readily – most of it is converted into water. However, a tiny proportion of the oxygen molecules are only partly converted and become so-called free radicals. These are oxygen atoms which contain unpaired electrons. In stable molecules all the electrons are paired. According to the rules of chemistry, unpaired electrons are desperate to find a partner. So oxygen-containing free radicals wreak havoc within the cell, tearing electrons from any molecule they happen to encounter – including proteins, DNA, and lipids (fat-soluble molecules including cholesterol).

When an oxygen-containing free radical does snatch an electron from a molecule, the oxygen atoms become attached to it in the process – leaving the molecule in what is known as an oxidised form. It has been estimated, for instance, that free radicals make around 100,000 hits a day on DNA. While DNA has a remarkable ability to repair itself, from time to time oxidative damage leads to mutation and the potential creation of a cancer (as we saw in Chapter 8). And, as we discussed in Chapter 5, oxidised low density lipoprotein is more likely to create atherosclerotic plaque, thereby laying the foundations for heart disease, than is the non-oxidised equivalent.

The body, however, has its own powerful defences against oxidation. Enzymes such as superoxide dismutase, glutathione peroxidase and catalase can disarm the free radicals by supplying them with electrons before they do any damage. But it is also known that vitamins A, C and E have powerful antioxidant effects. The evidence for this is overwhelming; in 120 out of 130 clinical studies people with high levels of vitamin C and E and beta-carotene (the precursor of vitamin A in the diet) in their blood had a lower risk of cancer than people with less of these vitamins.

Such evidence is the basis of official advice that we should eat at least five helpings of fruit and vegetables a day. Beta-carotene (an orange substance, as the name suggests) is found in highly coloured fruits and vegetables such as apricots, peppers, tomatoes, and – of course – carrots. Incidentally, evidence is mounting that lycopene, the chemical that gives tomatoes their red colour, is also a powerful antioxidant. Vitamin C is found in green leafy vegetables like spinach and in citrus fruits. The increasingly popular kiwi fruit is a very rich vitamin C source. Good sources of vitamin E include olives, vegetable and olive oil, avocadoes, and oily fish like mackerel and salmon. There are also significant antioxidants in tea, red wine, and spices such as turmeric, oregano and pepper. The minerals selenium and zinc – found in grains and fish, and oysters and muscle meat respectively – are also important antioxidants. They are components of antioxidant enzymes.

With so many dietary sources of antioxidants, surely supplementation must be unnecessary? Of course, people do not always eat the optimum diet – only a small percentage manage to consume the recommended five portions of fruit and vegetables. Recent surveys suggest that this is not due to lack of awareness, but arises from the stresses and pressures of everyday life which makes people opt out of breakfast or lunch and choose fast foods low in vitamin and mineral content.

There have been several clinical studies showing the benefits of supplements. One of the most recent, and most impressive, comes from the Cambridge Antioxidant Study (CHAOS). One of the members of this team was Malcolm Mitchison, who pioneered the idea that vitamin E may be helpful in preventing oxidation of lipids and the subsequent development of heart disease. In CHAOS, 2000 patients with atherosclerosis were studied. Half were put on 800 International Units (537 mg natural vitamin E) a day, while the rest were given a placebo. After 18 months, the vitamin E group had suffered only 25 per cent the number of heart attacks that had been suffered by the placebo group. Another study is underway in diabetic patients – a group which is particularly prone to heart disease. It has already been shown that vitamin E supplementation reduces LDL oxidation in these patients; what is currently lacking is information on how this translates into clinical outcome. Though no trials have yet been done, it is likely that vitamin E supplementation would have the most effect on patients with little, or no, sign of heart disease.

It is actually hard to get more than 50 mg a day of vitamin E from a normal diet. The RDA is still only 10 mg yet the amounts reckoned to give good protection against heart disease range from 60–100 mg. To get these amounts you would need to eat 55 grams of sunflower seeds, 170 grams of almonds, or 680 grams of peanut butter. The fat content of these foods is likely to put most people off consuming them in these quantities. So vitamin E presents itself as a genuine case for supplementation.

Clinical studies on beta-carotene have given conflicting results. Fifteen studies have shown that the higher the blood levels of beta-carotene, the lower the risk of lung cancer. But in a Swedish study of supplementation, people getting beta-carotene were actually 18 per cent *more* likely to develop lung cancer. Critics of this study have argued both that the subjects were high risk anyway, being heavy smokers, and that supplementation does not give the same beneficial effects as natural sources, such as carrots, which may contain other antioxidant substances.

Another antioxidant which may be in short supply – at least in the British diet – is selenium. Recommended amounts for a significant antioxidant effect are 50–60μg (there is currently no RDA). Sources include grains, fish and brazil nuts. Selenium is taken up from the soil, and there is concern that levels in British wheat may have declined in recent years leaving perhaps the majority of the population deficient in this important micronutrient.

However, in Europe and the US, the only officially sanctioned micronutrient supplement is folic acid. Four hundred μg a day is now recommended for women who intend to get pregnant after a number of studies showing that folic acid supplementation can prevent neural tube defects such as spina bifida in babies.

There is also good evidence that fatty acids in fish oils can help prevent heart disease, and that garlic aids the circulation and improves the elasticity of the arteries. Gammalinoleic acid in evening primrose oil is thought to be helpful in a number of conditions – from premenstrual syndrome and schizophrenia to arthritis and multiple sclerosis. However, whether people should improve their diet or spend money on these supplements remains an open scientific question.

There is another important issue. It has generally been assumed that substances found in the natural world are bound to be innocuous – despite centuries of evidence to the contrary (all the traditional toxins are natural products). Following on from this is an assumption that supplements can be sold without restriction. However, in the UK, there has been a recent move to limit the sale of vitamin B_6, which has prompted predictable outrage on the part of the health food industry.

Vitamin B_6 has been shown, by several clinical studies, to be helpful in the treatment of premenstrual syndrome when taken in amounts of 50–100 mg in the middle of the menstrual cycle. However, there has been one report – from 1987 – of neuropathy (pins and needles and numbness) in the limbs of people on doses as low as 50 mg. The effects were reversible on stopping the supplement, and the report has not been confirmed by subsequent studies. Nevertheless, the UK Government will only make 10 mg tablets freely available. This lower figure comes from dividing the supposed 'dangerous' upper limit of 50 mg by a safety margin of five. Amounts between 10–50 mg can only be obtained under the supervision of a pharmacist, while amounts greater than this are prescription only. Thus a food supplement has suddenly acquired the status of a pharmaceutical drug. Most experts in the field still argue that supplementation up to 200 mg a day is safe. It is tempting to wonder what all the fuss is about. If a genuine clinical condition such as PMS can be treated by vitamin B_6 and the evidence is convincing, then there is no reason why a doctor would not prescribe it – although they may not welcome the increased workload. It may well be that the vitamin B_6 decision is based on bad science (one clinical report not verified by independent research is a strong indication of bad science). It may be that the UK Government was looking for an opportunity to take on, and restrict, the activities of the supplements industry. If so, vitamin B_6 may turn out to be a poor vehicle for a long overdue attempt at regulation. In the meantime, more research into the effects of food supplements – particularly of antioxidants – must surely be merited, so we can decide whether the millions spent on supplements are justified.

Herbal medicines enter the mainstream

Herbs have, of course, been used as medicines for thousands of years. And, as we saw in Chapter 2, plant-based medicines still make a significant contribution to the pharmaceutical industry. According to the World Health Organization, 80 per cent of the world's population relies on traditional herbal medicines. They may be used almost exclusively, or – as in China – they may be integrated into modern medical practice. Elsewhere, as in Britain for instance, the use of herbal remedies is seen very much as an alternative to pharmaceutical drugs. However, there is increasing interest in herbal medicine in Europe – not least because of the example set by Germany where the herbal medicine industry is worth a massive $2 billion a year (ten times bigger than the UK market, and twice as large as that in the US).

Using extracts from leaves, flowers or seeds is vastly different from adminstering a pharmaceutical drug. Herbal extracts may contain hundreds of active compounds, while the pharmaceutical drug usually contains only one. Herbalists argue that the presence of many active ingredients is beneficial, for they can act in a synergistic way (in other words, the whole is greater than the sum of the parts). But the complexity of plant extracts renders herbalism a rather inexact science. The concentration of active ingredients is likely to vary with the source of the plant material, and with the time of gathering. The composition of the medicine may also depend upon the way it is prepared, stored and handled. However, many companies are now developing technologies for manufacturing herbal remedies with standardised and guaranteed concentrations of active ingredients.

The chemistry and pharmacology of the active ingredients of herbal medicines have been researched for many years. There are major studies underway of the herbal medicines of China, Japan, and India at Harvard, London and Exeter Universities. And botanists at London's Kew Gardens are planning a major collection of Chinese medicinal plants, which will be the first to be created outside China. What has been lacking has been reliable, reproducible clinical trials on the efficacy of these remedies, which could allow them to take their place alongside more conventional medicines. However, this may change; thirteen major drug companies are said to be buying up or entering collaborations with manufacturers of herbal remedies.

Herbs for the mind? Hypericum and ginkgo

Two remedies which are especially popular in Germany – hypericum and ginkgo – are backed by a reasonable body of scientific research. These may be joined by many more if the current interest in herbal medicine is sustained.

Hypericum is an extract from the yellow flowers of *Hypericum perforatum* or St John's Wort, so called because it blooms around the birthday of St John the Baptist–June 24th. The plant grows on heathland and in woods in Europe, Western Asia, and North Africa. Hypericum has been used medically for around 2000 years, and was described by the physician Paracelsus (1493–1541). In the Middle Ages, physicians used it against 'dreadful melancholic thoughts' or 'to drive out the Devil'. In other words, hypericum is traditionally known as an anti-depressant, although it has many other uses – such as wound healing. Today it is used very extensively in Germany, where 66 million daily doses were taken in 1994, at a cost of £26 million. In Germany, a herbal remedy can get a marketing authorisation using a specific monograph for the plant which takes the place of the registration dossier that would be produced for a pharmaceutical drug. In 1984, such a monograph identified the major active ingredient as hypericin, and described it as having monoamine oxidase inhibitor properties. Subsequent research has suggested that there may be much more to hypericum's anti-depressant and anxiolytic effect than this; the hypericin molecule also resembles a tricyclic anti-depressant in its chemical structure and in some of its pharmacological actions.

Unusually for a herbal medicine, hypericum has been subject to many clinical trials. Edzard Ernst, the UK's first ever professor of complementary medicine at Exeter University, reviewed the data available in 1995. He found eight high quality random double-blinded clinical trials of hypericin against placebo, and three against standard anti-depressant drugs such as imipramine. His study concluded that hypericin is better than placebo, and about as good as imipramine in relieving mild to moderate depression. It relieves a wide variety of depression-related symptoms, such as anxiety, insomnia, headache and exhaustion. A real bonus is that people on hypericin experience far fewer side effects than they do on tricyclics. So, even if the anti-depressant effect is about the same, in real terms hypericin could be more effective because patients are more likely to keep taking it for the few weeks necessary before its beneficial effects kick in.

A recent trial by David Wheatley of the Royal Masonic Hospital in London trialled hypericin against amitriptyline and found it to be equally effective. And there have been many less formal, smaller and open studies which showed similar effects. For instance, at the launch of hypericin in tablet form in the UK, 146 members of the general population took the supplement for two weeks. When surveyed 75 per cent said they felt better in the morning, 67 per cent were enjoying a better sex life, and 33 per cent claimed to be better able to deal with criticism. This supplement, which is on general sale, contains 300 µg hypericin per tablet, which is much less concentrated than the tincture prescribed for depression in Germany. The supplement, known as Kira, is marketed with the careful wording 'could help to maintain your emotional balance and well being'. It is the first over-the-counter anti-depressant.

More recent studies have suggested that hypericin is effective for seasonal affective disorder and menopausal depression. But many psychiatrists are calling for more study of hypericin before it is licensed more widely as an anti-depressant. They say that patient groups have been too diverse in many of the studies to date, and there is little information on whether hypericin is effective in severe depression.

The other herbal remedy which has been the subject of much study is ginkgo. This comes from the tree *Ginkgo biloba* or the maidenhair tree – so called because of the resemblance of the shape of its leaves to those of the maidenhair fern. Charles Darwin described the Ginkgo tree as a living fossil, because it is the only living member of the order of plants called the gymnosperms. These flourished in the Jurassic Age – along with dinosaurs – 150 million years ago, but were overtaken by flowering plants and conifers. It grows wild in China, and is widely cultivated. It has long been sacred in the Far East, and is planted in Buddhist temples and palaces. In China, ginkgo has been used for 5000 years and is revered as a remedy that brings wisdom.

Ginkgo extract improves circulation to the brain, and to the limbs. It has been shown to improve cognitive functions such as memory, alertness and concentration in both healthy volunteers and in people with dementia. It also helps with Raynaud's syndrome, a painful condition in which circulation to the fingers is impaired, and with many other circulatory conditions.

There are three classes of active ingredient in ginkgo – flavonoids, ginkgolides and bilobalides. The flavonoids, as we saw in the last section, are potent antioxidants and so may prevent age-related brain dysfunction by preventing oxidative damage to cells. They are also – like aspirin – inhibitors of cyclooxygenase (see also Chapter 1) and so may thin the blood, making it flow more readily. The ginkgolides inhibit a molecule called platelet activating factor (PAF), which is a specific trigger for inflammation. It is possible that inflammation plays a role in brain dysfunction. Gingko is also being trialled for asthma; it is known that PAF plays a role in sensitising and narrowing the airways in response to asthma triggers. Inhibition of PAF could also be important in treating stroke and burns. The bilobalides appear to help regrowth of neurons, as well as limiting the damage caused by cerebral ischaemia (impairment of the oxygen supply to the brain).

Melatonin, the darkness hormone

In the case of melatonin, public opinion has far outstripped clinical data, thanks largely to two popular books extolling the virtues of this natural hormone. In *The Melatonin Miracle*, Walter Pierpaoli and William Regelson claim it prevents ageing, while Russel Reiter and Jo Robinson's book *Melatonin:your body's wonder drug*, makes much of is antioxidant properties (it is said to be more potent than vitamins C or E). However, all the clinical studies to date have been on melatonin's effect on disorders of the human sleep–wake cycle.

Melatonin is produced by the pea-sized pineal gland in the centre of the brain as a response to falling light levels perceived by the retina of the eye – thus, it is known as the darkness hormone. It was discovered in 1958 by Aaron Lerner of Yale University, who found that it could lighten the skin of frogs. Because it affects structures in frog skin cells that produce the pigment melanin (which is also responsible for the colour of human skin and hair) he named it melatonin.

Blood levels of melatonin wax and wane during the night. In the small hours, levels would be typically 80 parts per billion, falling to 10 parts per billion just before dawn. The secretion of melatonin organises sleep–wake cycles in humans and other mammals. The exact mode of action of melatonin is not fully understood, but it acts on receptors in the body's internal clock, the superchiasmic nuclei (SCN) which is situated behind the eyes, and causes drowsiness, fall in body temperature and other physiological changes associated with sleep.

Human sleep–wake cycles are strongly tied – through the melatonin/SCN mechanism – to the external environment. Since we are diurnal animals (unlike bats, for instance, which are nocturnal) we are generally awake when it is light and asleep when it is dark. However, Josephine Arendt, a leading melatonin researcher at the University of Surrey, has shown that adminstering small amounts of the hormone to humans can advance or delay the sleep–wake cycle.

There is an obvious application here; melatonin could help people retune sleep–wake cycles which have fallen out of sync with the external environment – such as people with jet lag, shift workers, and the blind. For instance, if you travel across several time zones from west to east (from the US to the UK, say), the external clock will advance by five hours more than your internal clock. So your body may tell you it is 6 pm – long before bedtime – when it is 11 pm outside. This results in jet lag – inability to sleep at bedtime, followed by daytime sleepiness. Shift workers have to be alert, when their internal clock is telling them it is bedtime, and often suffer from similar problems. And over half of blind people surveyed had sleep disturbances due to their lack of environmental light–dark cues.

Studies carried out by Arendt and others have shown that melatonin, given at the right time, can either advance or delay the onset of sleep, therefore effectively 'retuning' the sleep–wake cycle. In practical terms, melatonin can relieve jet lag, as shown by studies on nearly 500 air travellers. Smaller studies have shown that it is helpful for shift workers and blind people. However, there is little evidence for the claims that it helps cure cancer, AIDS, Alzheimer's disease and high blood pressure. And while it is true that levels of melatonin do fall with age, Pierpaoli and Regelson's anti-ageing claims are based upon animal experiments of doubtful relevance to humans.

Melatonin is freely available in the United States, where it is said to be more popular than aspirin. But in the UK, it can only be obtained on prescription. The recent reclassification, imposed by the Medicines Control Agency (MCA) led to dramatic seizures by enforcement officers of the agency, rumours of 'under-the-counter' sales to desperate customers, and caseloads of the hormone being brought back illicitly from the US. The restriction was based on concerns that, as a hormone, melatonin has power-ful physiological effects which have been insufficiently studied and that it should be licensed as a drug, rather than as a food supplement.

Certainly there is now an urgent need for long-term study as melatonin is being consumed so widely in the US. The manufacturers have challenged the MCA's ban – arguing, predictably, that melatonin is 'natural' because it occurs in bananas and tomatoes. However, the amounts consumed in supplements are far higher than those which occur in the average diet. If the manufacturers, Pharma Nord, win their appeal, we could see wider sale of other natural products which are currently available on prescription only – and this move would be a great triumph for the health foods and natural medicines industry. Meanwhile, at least three pharmaceutical com-panies are developing melatonin analogues.

Herbal hazards

The legal status of herbal remedies varies between countries. Some are treated as food supplements (as are vitamins and minerals), while others can be sold as medicines, if certain criteria are met. In the UK and the US, herbal remedies can only become a licensed drug if they are backed by the same level of knowledge on safety and efficacy as a conventional pharma-ceutical drug. Elsewhere, as in Germany for instance, the regulations are less stringent. However, the net result is that most herbal remedies are sold and used outside the controls which apply to pharmaceutical drugs. So it seems reasonable to ask whether they pose any risk to human health. To say that all natural products are harmless is naive. Biologically active chemicals derive their mode of action ultimately from their chemical structure, not from their source. So it follows that benign chemicals can be made in a lab, and potent toxins can occur in nature. Luckily, most herbal remedies have a long tradition of human use and we can, in most cases, rely on this knowl-edge to feel pretty safe in using them. Where we are probably most vulner-able, in the West, is in our use of imported remedies of which our under-standing is limited.

The Medical Toxicology Unit of Guy's Hospital, London, has recently completed a five year survey of adverse effects associated with food sup-plements and unlicensed herbal remedies. They found a link between prod-ucts and ill health in 12 cases. Of these, nine related to the use of Indian remedies which contain toxic heavy metals such as lead, arsenic and mercury. One case involved poisoning from a Chinese remedy, another was a case of liver failure from copper tablets, while the final one involved development high blood pressure from taking ginseng for several years.

There have been several other cases of liver failure reported from Chinese herbal remedies around the world – particularly with treatments for AIDS. This is worrying, as shops selling these remedies are springing up all around the UK. While no one is disputing the potential value of these medicines (one is already under development as a treatment for eczema, which works where conventional treatment has failed), they are really in quite a different league from garlic supplements or camomile tea. They are complex mixtures, containing ingredients that few Westerners are familiar with, and should really only be taken under the supervision of a qualified practitioner.

But there have also been problems with herbs that are well known in Europe. Comfrey, a common hairy perennial with distinctive blue and pink flowers, has long been used for a wide range of purposes, from sleeping aid to wound healer. In fact, it contains toxic compounds called pyrrolizidine alkaloids which can damage the liver. Remedies based on comfrey have been banned in several countries. Other herbs with possible toxic effects include pennyroyal, germander and sassafras.

There have also been several deaths linked to the use of herbal remedies containing the stimulant ephedrine (which, as we saw in the last chapter, is related to amphetamine). These have been marketed as a safe alternative to Ecstasy under the names Herbal Ecstasy, Cloud 9, and Ultimate Xphoria. Ephedrine causes an increase in heart rate and blood pressure which, in susceptible individuals, progresses to a heart attack or a stroke. In the US, the Food and Drug Administration has issued a formal warning about Herbal Ecstasy, but has stopped short of an outright ban. In the UK, the MCA stepped in shortly after Herbal Ecstasy hit the dance clubs and made it illegal to sell it without a licence, effectively stamping out the drug's use.

However, for all the publicity they generate, hazards from herbs are rare. According to the American Association of Poison Control Centres, you are five hundred times more likely to be killed by a pharmaceutical drug than by a herbal remedy.

It is likely that the use of herbal medicines will grow, given the public interest in complementary medicine. But the major future trend with pharmaceutical drugs will be the introduction of gene-based medicine – the subject of the next, and final, chapter.

11

In the pipeline: gene-based medicine

The future of the pharmaceutical industry is certain to be shaped by gene-based medicine (or genomics, as it is often called). Francis Crick and James Watson, co-discoverers of the structure of the DNA molecule in 1953, were insightful enough to see that their discovery would have a major impact on the understanding of how cells work. But it is doubtful if they then appreciated the practical potential of their discovery for human health (although Watson was, until recently, director of the Human Genome Project, whose implications for drug development we will discuss below).

DNA is the chemical which genes are made from, and it occurs within the nucleus of every cell in the body. It is a polymeric molecule, made of four types of repeating chemical units called nucleotides. These, in turn, are formed of three chemical parts – a phosphate group, a molecule of a sugar called ribose, and a base, which is a small molecule containing one or more nitrogen atoms. It is the base which varies; there are four types of base in DNA – adenine, guanine, cytosine and thymine (often abbreviated to A, G, C and T).

Crick and Watson showed that the DNA molecule consists of two separate strands wound around one another in a double helix. The phosphate groups are on the outside, while the bases face one another in pairs in the centre of the helix, joined together by weak chemical bonds known as hydrogen bonds (A always pairs with T and G with C). The ribose groups bridge the phosphates and the bases (see Fig. 11.1).

The bases – three billion of them in a single strand of human DNA – are arranged in apparently random order, e.g. AATCGTATA ... In 1961, Crick and others discovered the genetic code buried within this sequence. If you call each base symbol a 'letter', then there are 64 possible three letter 'words' (ATA, AGA and so on), each known as a codon.

If you 'read' a DNA sequence in terms of codons, segments of it make

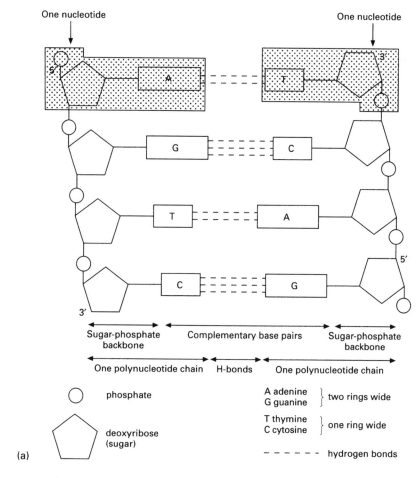

(a)

Fig. 11.1. The structure of DNA. (a) Structure of DNA represented as two 'straightened' paired chains. Each nucleotide unit in the DNA molecule is made up of three parts: phosphate, sugar and base. These bases pair together by hydrogen bonding down the centre of the two chains – A with T and C with G. (b) The DNA double helix. The DNA molecule consists of two long chains twisted around one another to make a double helix.

biochemical sense. Working around the time of Crick and his colleagues, Marshall Nirenberg and Johann Matthei at the National Institutes of Health in Washington broke the code, showing that each codon corresponded to a different amino acid. Segments of DNA, known as genes, correspond to the amino acid sequences of the thousands of proteins which are needed to carry

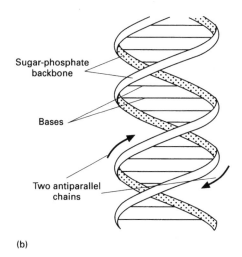

Sugar-phosphate backbone

Bases

Two antiparallel chains

(b)

Fig. 11.1. *cont'd.*

out the biochemical activities of cells. Most of these proteins are enzymes – catalysing reactions as varied as the extraction of energy from glucose to the creation of neurotransmitters from simpler chemicals. Other proteins are the stuff our bodies are made of – actin in muscle, collagen in skin and keratin in hair and nails, for instance.

There are between 50,000 and 100,000 different genes, encoding the amino acid sequences of different proteins, within the human DNA molecule. In fact this only accounts for one to two per cent of the three billion nucleotides making up the molecule (the function of the rest is one of the most fascinating mysteries in modern biology, but is unfortunately outside the scope of this book).

After the discovery of the genetic code, it took several more years before researchers found just how protein molecules were created from the genes that code for them. The basic features of this important process are outlined in Fig. 11.2 (and have already been discussed briefly in the context of the mode of action of antibiotics in Chapter 3). First the two strands are opened up, by the action of an enzyme called RNA polymerase, and one strand (known as the antisense or template strand) is copied in a process called transcription. The copy is not DNA, but a related molecule called RNA (ribonucleic acid). The slight chemical differences between RNA and DNA are that the base uracil (U) stands in for thymine, and the sugar ribose for deoxyribose – but these differences are not particularly relevant to our

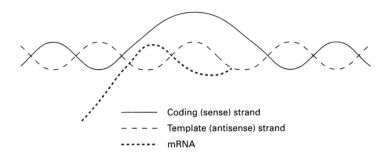

———— Coding (sense) strand
– – – – Template (antisense) strand
······· mRNA

Fig. 11.2. Transcription of DNA. The enzyme RNA polymerase opens up the double helix of DNA, seen in the centre of the diagram, so that the template (antisense) strand of DNA can be copied into messenger RNA (mRNA). Complementary bases line up during transcription – therefore mRNA has the same sequence of the coding (sense) strand DNA (except that the base uracil stands in for the base thymine).

discussion here. The RNA copy of a gene made during its transcription is called messenger RNA, or mRNA.

Transcription occurs in the nucleus of a cell, but the mRNA drifts out into the cytoplasm to a structure known as a ribosome (itself made of another type of RNA) where the message it bears is 'read' and translated into a protein molecule of the correct amino acid sequence (Fig. 11.3). Central to this process is an 'adaptor' molecule known as transfer RNA (tRNA). This contains a three base sequence called an anticodon which is complementary to that of a particular codon. To the other end is attached the amino acid for that particular codon. When the anticodon homes in on its codon on the mRNA strand, it brings the appropriate amino acid into line. Once the whole mRNA molecule is 'read', a corresponding protein molecule, with the correct amino acid sequence, can be assembled.

What has any of this got to do with making new drugs? There are many potential applications from these ground-breaking discoveries in the field of DNA technology. Transferring human genes to other species by genetic engineering techniques allows the production of human proteins in large quantities and some of these are completely new drugs. It is also possible to use DNA itself as a drug – either to turn off the activity of genes during disease states or, ultimately, as genes which will either replace those which are faulty or missing, or as production units to make useful

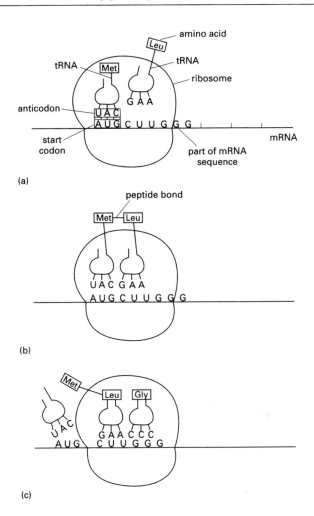

Fig. 11.3. Translation of mRNA into protein. (a) tRNAs, loaded with amino acids, move into position on the ribosome as codon–anticodon pairs are formed (the abbreviations Met, Leu and Gly refer to different amino acids). (b) A chemical bond, called a peptide bond, is formed between two amino acids. (c) Protein assembly continues as loaded tRNAs drift away, and the next amino acid moves into position.

proteins within the body. And of course, the more we know about the working of our genes, the more precise and effective new medicines can be.

Genetic engineering for new pharmaceuticals

With genetic engineering, a gene for a human protein can be transferred to another species which will treat the gene as one of its own, turning out copies of the appropriate molecule which can then be isolated and purified as a medicine. The first medicine to be produced in this way was human insulin, in 1982 (Fig. 11.4). The DNA for human insulin was transferred into a 'circle' of bacterial DNA called a plasmid, using specific enzymes to make the appropriate chemical bonds. The nice thing about plasmid DNA, is that it enters 'host' bacterial cells quite naturally, and so acts as a shuttle (or vector, to use the technical term) carrying human insulin DNA into *E. coli* bacteria. These now treat the insulin gene as one of their own, and if grown in a fermenter they will turn out lots of copies of human insulin molecules, which can then be separated and purified.

Until the advent of human insulin, diabetics had to rely on insulin extracted from pig or cattle pancreas. These differ by a few amino acids from human insulin and occasionally cause allergic reactions in patients. And, as we now know to our cost, extracting drugs from animal – including human – tissue poses an ever-present risk of contamination. Growth hormone was traditionally prepared from pituitary glands collected from mortuaries by technicians paid a nominal sum for the task. Occasionally, a gland was taken from someone suffering from Creuzfeldt-Jakob disease (the human form of BSE) and infection was passed on through the growth hormone. Thousands of haemophiliacs became infected with HIV after receiving the clotting Factor VIII extracted from contaminated blood in the 1980s. Thanks to genetic engineering, the danger of infection from these products is over. Protein drugs produced by genetic engineering are known as recombinant drugs or therapeutic proteins. A list of those currently on the market is given in Table 3; by the year 2000 there will be an estimated 100 therapeutic proteins available. These are being developed against cancer, AIDS, asthma, diabetes, rheumatism, mutliple sclerosis, stroke, viral infections and wound healing.

The exciting thing about therapeutic proteins is that several are genuinely innovative drugs. Interferon-β – although controversial – is the first real

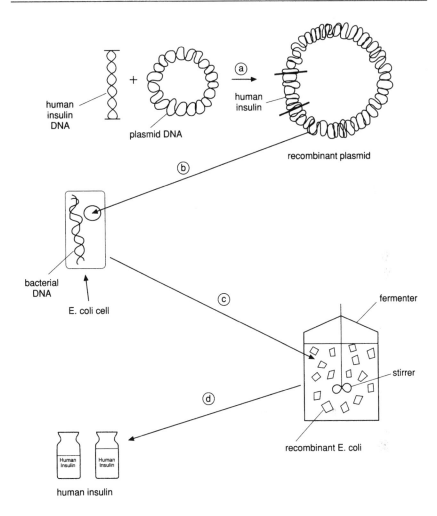

Fig. 11.4. Production of human insulin by genetic engineering. The DNA of the human insulin gene is mixed with bacterial plasmid DNA and an enzyme, creating a recombinant DNA plasmid (a). This is transferred into *E. coli* bacteria (b). The recombinant bacteria are then grown in a fermenter (c) where they manufacture human insulin. This is extracted and purified to make pure human insulin (d).

drug for multiple sclerosis. Erythropoietin (EPO) is a hormone produced by the kidneys which helps create new red blood cells. Its synthesis is impaired in kidney failure and so such patients generally require repeated blood transfusions; this impairs their quality of life, exposes them to the

Table 3. *Therapeutic proteins currently on the market*

Product name	Use
Humulin (human insulin)	Diabetes
Protropin (human growth hormone)[a]	Dwarfism
Intron A (interferon)[b]	Leukaemia
Roferon A (interferon)	Leukaemia
Recombivax (hepatitis B vaccine)	Prevention of hepatitis B
Humatrope (human growth hormone)	Dwarfism
Activase (tissue plasminogen activator)	Heart attack
EPOGEN (erythropoietin)	Anaemia in kidney disease
Engerix B (hepatitis B vaccine)	Prevention of hepatitis B
Alferon N (interferon)	Genital warts
Actimmune (interferon)	Chronic granulomatosis[c]
NEUPOGEN (colony stimulating factor)[d]	Chemotherapy-induced neutropenia[e]
Leukin (colony stimulating factor)	Bone marrow transplantation
Proleukin (interleukin-2)	Kidney cancer
Recombinate (antihaemophilic factor)	Haemophilia
KoGENate (Factor VIII)	Haemophilia
Betaseron (interferon)	Multiple sclerosis
Pulmozyme (DNAse)[f]	Cystic fibrosis
Nutropin (somatotropin)[g]	Growth failure in children with kidney problems
Cerezyme (glucocerebrosidase)[h]	Gaucher's disease (i)

[a]There are two forms of growth hormone and two forms of hepatitis B vaccine made by different companies

[b]There are several forms of interferon, each with a different clinical application

[c]A disorder of the white blood cells occurring in many diseases eg tuberculosis

[d]A growth factor which stimulates the production of white blood cells

[e]The fall in white blood cell count which occurs as a result of anti-cancer drugs attacking the stem cells in the bone marrow

[f]An enzyme which breaks down DNA of bacteria causing lung infections

[g]A growth hormone

[h]An enzyme which breaks down cerebrosides, compounds deposited around nerve fibres

[i]A genetic disease characterised by lack of the enzyme described in (h) and abnormal deposits of cerebroside in various parts of the body

(admittedly minimal) risk of infection, and risks iron overload, which is toxic to the heart. So far 100,000 kidney patients worldwide are benefiting from EPO, which allows them to do without transfusions. It is also useful for anaemia which occurs in AIDS patients.

Antibodies are another important group of therapeutic proteins. As we saw in Chapter 3, these are produced by the body in response to an external threat, such as an invading microbe. Molecules on the surface of a 'foreign' substance like a microbe, called antigens, elicit the full firepower of the immune system – part of which is the production of antibodies which stick to the antigen and label the invader for destruction by white blood cells. Antibodies can be created from the appropriate genes by genetic engineering and used in therapeutic roles other than combatting infection. They can neutralise the action of individual molecules in the body (rather than complete microbes). Monoclonal antibodies have been tried, with little success, in septic shock, where they failed to damp down the inflammatory process to a great enough extent. However, they show much more promise in another inflammatory condition, rheumatoid arthritis. In a recent phase II trial of an antibody against tumour necrosis factor, a key molecule in inflammation, 75 per cent of patients showed significant improvement in their arthritis, compared to only 14 per cent in a placebo group. Others monoclonal antibodies are being trialled against some of the molecules of the immune system which are produced in response to organ transplants as part of the rejection process; if these could be 'silenced' then the graft would have more chance of settling down in the recipient's body.

Recombinant vaccines are also an important new group of therapeutic agents. Two brands of a vaccine against hepatitis B are already in general use; those in development are naturally occurring protein antigens which will hopefully elicit a strong immune response without the problems of using 'live' virus bearing these antigens (the so-called dirty vaccines).

And, besides innovation, recombinant drugs offer other advantages to both patients and pharmaceutical companies. So far they seem to get to the marketplace faster than conventional small molecule drugs. They are, on the whole, less toxic because they are naturally produced in the body. And there is enormous potential to produce them very cheaply.

So far most recombinant drugs have been produced using cells in fermenters. The bacterium *E. coli* is good at producing relatively simple proteins such as insulin. However, for more complex proteins such as antibodies or blood clotting factors it has been necessary to move to cells which are more like human cells. Only these possess the biochemical machinery to fold up the recombinant protein molecules into their correct functional shape. And many protein molecules get small sugar molecules added to them after synthesis, in a process known as glycosylation. Bacterial cells do not carry out glycosylation, but without it a protein could be rendered useless. So yeast, insect, and mammalian cells – such as Chinese hamster ovary (CHO) cells – have all been pressed into service for the manufacture of therapeutic proteins. But these cells all have to be cultured – turning out therapeutic protein molecules as they grow and multiply – in vast, stainless steel fermenters, which must be kept sterilised at all costs and are computer controlled for temperature, acidity and nutrient level. Such fermentations can work out expensive. So there has been a move, in recent years, towards the use of living bioreactors.

Few of you reading this will have been untouched by the excitement surrounding the creation of Dolly, the cloned sheep. To recap, the DNA from a sheep's udder cell was transferred to a donor egg from which the nucleus had been removed. The egg was then transferred to a surrogate mother and the embryo developed into Dolly – who is, more or less, an identical genetic copy of her mother (more or less because there is DNA in mitochondria, outside the nucleus, and this was not transferred from the udder cell). The main point about creating Dolly, which might have been missed in all the hype about the possibility of human cloning, is that the project was meant to point the way to more efficient and cost-effective ways of producing human proteins in sheep milk.

To backtrack a little, scientists at the Roslin Institute in Edinburgh (whose commercial spin-off is the company PPL) have long been interested in the transfer of human genes to sheep, targetted to produce the relevant protein in their milk. They create the transgenic animals (transgenic meaning bearing a foreign gene – in this case a human gene) by transferring the gene to a fertilised sheep egg, by injection. The eggs are transferred to surrogate mothers for gestation. It is quite an inefficient process as it stands; only a few per cent of the sheep born from this process bear the human gene and produce the relevant protein in their milk. Nevertheless, PPL already has a flock of sheep which are producing a human protein called α-1 anti-trypsin (AAT). This inhibits the enzyme elastase (actually a close relative of trypsin), which digests lung tissue under certain pathological conditions such as emphysema and cystic fibrosis (CF). AAT is now in phase II trials in CF, an inherited lung disorder which affects 55,000 people in the US and Europe – being the commonest inherited disorder in these areas. With cloned sheep like Dolly, cells could be manipulated in the laboratory until it was known that the gene had been taken up (instead of waiting until an animal was born) and that cell's DNA transferred to an egg cell. In a second line of attack, transgenic animals known to produce high levels of human proteins could be cloned, producing an elite flock. Such cloning would make the whole transgenic production process more predictable, cheaper, and quicker, and would use fewer animals.

Transgenic animals such as pigs, sheep, cattle, and rabbits are being used to produce a wide range of therapeutic proteins in their milk. But it is also possible to produce such proteins in plants too (sidestepping animal welfare problems). Plants have shown they are very good at soaking up new DNA – the main problems have, to date, been in growing on crops of such plants. The signs are that antibodies and vaccines will be produced very cheaply in plants such as tobacco in the near future.

And just as chemists tinker with the structure of small molecule drugs to enhance their performance, so genetic engineers can improve therapeutic proteins. By altering the genetic code (changing an A for a T, for example, or even by deleting whole chunks of the code) and then transferring the new version of the gene to the appropriate bioreactor, altered (or 'engineered') versions of the original protein can be created. These may turn out to be more useful than the natural proteins, which are not necessarily optimised for therapeutic use.

Protein engineering has already been used to create new versions of the clot-busting drug tissue plasminogen activator (tPA), whose therapeutic action was discussed in Chapter 5. Natural tPA has a short lifetime in the body, which means it has to be continuously infused. The tPA molecule is composed of five functional regions, one of which binds to the fibrin clot while another has the enzyme-like activity which dissolves it. Reteplase, an engineered version, is a far smaller molecule containing only the two domains which have been found essential to its activity. Therefore it has a longer lifetime in the body, which means it is easier to administer – as just two single injections. Since it lacks the domain that actually sticks to the clot, Reteplase may actually be more effective, because its molecules are free to permeate the clot and dissolve it from inside.

The latest results from the GUSTO (short for Global Use of STrategies to Open occluded arteries) trial – which is trying to evaluate the best way to treat people after heart attacks, show little difference between tPA and Reteplase. Thirty days after a heart attack, only seven per cent of the 15,000 plus patients in the trial had died – on either drug. Where Reteplase is likely to score clinically is in its ease of administration (a vital

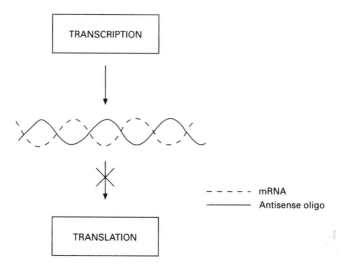

Fig. 11.5. How antisense oligos work. Transcription produces a single strand of mRNA which would normally go through to translation. However, a complementary strand of antisense DNA will create a double helix, as shown, which cannot he translated, so gene expression is turned off. Note that the oligo must have the same sequence as the antisense or template strand of the original DNA; it is complementary to the mRNA which, in turn, was complementary to this strand of DNA.

factor in a busy intensive care unit). The genetic engineers will not stop at Reteplase: there are already many more engineered versions of tPA in the pipeline.

Making sense of antisense

In 1978, Paul Zamecnik of Harvard University demonstrated that the DNA to protein machinery could be interrupted by the use of small synthetic stretches of DNA called oligonucleotides (oligos for short). He used an oligo with a sequence complementary to an mRNA molecule which Rous sarcoma virus (which causes tumours in chickens) needs to reproduce itself. This oligo bound to the mRNA and so stopped it moving on to the ribosome for translation. Such oligos are known as antisense oligos, because they have the same sequence as the antisense or template strand of the corresponding DNA (see Fig. 11.5).

Now Zamecnik's brilliant idea is being transformed into a range of specific DNA drugs against cancer, viral infection and Crohn's disease (an inflammatory condition of the bowel). By turning off the expression of genes active in disease, the oligos nip the disorder in the bud or stop its progress (so the theory goes). After some technical problems during the early development stages, there are now 12 antisense drugs well on their way. In leukaemia, for example, Alan Gewirtz at the University of Pennsylvania has treated 15 patients with chronic myelogenous leukaemia by removing some of their bone marrow and exposing it to an antisense oligo against a gene called *c-myb*. This is just one of the many genes involved in abnormal cell division (see also Chapter 7). Turning it off in these patients had a dramatic effect; once the treated bone marrow was returned to their body, their remission rates increased by 50 per cent. Better still they experienced no toxic side effects (compare that to the suffering that conventional cancer chemotherapy causes).

There are two small US biotech companies which specialised in antisense drugs – Isis and Hybridon. It seems likely that a drug created by Isis, fomivirsen, which treats the cytomegalovirus infections occurring in AIDS, will be the first drug of this type on the market; it is currently doing well in phase III clinical trials.

If there is a major problem with recombinant and antisense drugs, it is in how to deliver them to their targets. Currently, proteins cannot be taken by mouth because they will be digested in the gut before they reach the bloodstream. Even in the blood, they may be degraded by enzymes before entering cells. And as large molecules, they do not diffuse through cell membranes in the way small, conventional, drug molecules do. Instead they are taken in by a process called exocytosis, in which the membrane folds in on itself to form a small cavity which then engulfs the protein molecule, taking it into the cytoplasm. All these problems currently mean that high doses have to be given to allow therapeutic doses to reach their target – which pushes costs up. However, new developments in inhalation technology for drug delivery (see also the discussion on drug delivery in Chapter 2) promises to make recombinant drugs a more practical and affordable option in the near future. Many of the same problems apply to oligos, which are also quite a bit larger than conventional drug molecules. These have to be delivered to the nucleus of the cell, which is where they act on mRNA. With oligos, which are synthetic – rather than recombinant – molecules, the delivery problems may be addressed by modifying the chemistry of the drug molecules.

The promise of gene therapy

When people talk about DNA and medicine, they will always mention gene therapy – far more than recombinant drugs, or developments such as anti-sense therapy. Which is odd in one way, because it will be well into the 21st century before gene therapy is generally available. Maybe the prospect of gene therapy attracts so much interest – and controversy – because it really is a radical departure for the pharmaceutical industry. In gene therapy, the genome (the name given to all the genetic material) of an individual will be altered. In a sense, patients are given the means of making their own drug; instead of taking a tablet which has been made in a factory, they are given a gene which will make the protein which is the drug. So in one sense, it is just using the patients themselves as bioreactors.

However, tinkering with people's genes obviously cannot be done lightly. A fundamental distinction between two types of gene therapy needs to be made at this point. We have two types of cells in our bodies. Germ cells – sperm and egg – carry genes to the next generation, while all the other cells, which are known as somatic cells, die with the individual. Germ cell gene therapy would possibly carry the new genes on through the generations, while somatic cell gene therapy would be only for the individual during his or her lifetime. At this stage, no one is talking about germ line gene therapy (although they will, in the future, without doubt). So all the possibilities we will discuss here relate only to somatic gene therapy.

The scope of gene therapy is actually now quite broad. Originally the concept was fairly simple; gene therapy would be applied to patients suffering from single-gene disorders such as cystic fibrosis or haemophilia. The new gene would take over the function of the missing or faulty gene. There are over 5000 of these single-gene disorders and, it has to be said, most of them are quite rare. Cystic fibrosis is the commonest in the Western world, affecting one in 2000 children born. There would be obvious financial barriers to developing gene therapies for the very rare diseases.

However, more recently it has been proposed that gene therapy could be applied to any disease that has a genetic component. This broadens its scope enormously to include cancer, heart disease, neurological disease and even infections such as AIDS, with the idea being to deliver genes that would make therapeutic proteins – altering the genome in such a way as to help the body fight the disease.

The technology of gene therapy is broadly similar to the genetic engineering process described in Fig. 11.4 and can be divided into three stages –

getting the gene required, putting it into a vector, and delivering it to the right place. It is these last two stages which are particularly tricky in human gene therapy. In other words, the choice of vector to shuttle the gene into the body is crucial, and getting the gene to function correctly within the body is a problem peculiar to human gene therapy.

Many different types of vector have been developed – and it is becoming increasingly obvious that the choice of vector depends very much on what you want the gene therapy to do. Viruses were the first vectors to be investigated. It might sound risky to subject people to viral infection as part of a therapeutic programme. But viruses have a natural ability to get inside human cells and if they are loaded up with therapeutic genes, then they should take the genes to their target cell. And viruses can be manipulated by adding and subtracting genes to make them harmless (although there is no absolute guarantee that they will not revert, at some stage, to virulence).

The retroviruses, which have RNA not DNA in their genome, have long been favoured as vehicles for gene therapy because they are able to integrate the new genes into the chromosomes of the cell, so that they stay there long-term, making one-off treatment for a genetic disorder a distinct possibility. But they only enter dividing cells, which – so far – limits their application. And there is also a concern that they could insert the new gene into the wrong place in a chromosome and either inactivate some vital gene which is already there, or even trigger activity in a cancer gene present at the insertion site. Research into the creation of new retroviruses which can enter a wider range of cells is, however, ongoing – as is study of ways of inserting them more precisely into the chromosome. It may sound incredible, but HIV is being tested as a gene therapy vector as it is a retrovirus which infects non-dividing cells. It is being engineered to make it innocuous, but the authorities are understandably nervous about the safety of any clinical trials arising from this work.

An alternative viral vector is the adenovirus – otherwise known as the common cold virus. This is probably safer, from the point of view of infection, than are the retroviruses. It deposits its gene cargo outside the chromosome, and over time this may be lost. So patients having gene therapy with adenovirus vectors may need the treatment repeated – for cystic fibrosis, say. However, one treatment may be sufficient to treat a tumour with genes that stimulate the immune system.

The herpes virus, which causes cold sores, chicken pox and shingles, has a special affinity for neurons and so is being trialled for neurological problems such as brain tumours and Parkinson's disease.

Better still, from a safety point of view, are the adeno-associated viruses, which do not cause disease in man, and have the added advantage of inserting genes into the chromosome – like the retroviruses. But there are also non-viral vectors, which eliminate the risk of infection altogether.

Chief among these are the liposomes. These are fatty droplets in which DNA – the genes to be delivered – can be wrapped in the form of a plasmid. Liposomes have already been used in aerosol form as a vector in advanced clinical trials of gene therapy for both cystic fibrosis and cancer. It is even possible to get 'naked' DNA into cells – doing away with the need for a vector altogether. This technology promises to be very useful for the development of vaccines. The idea is that the gene – or perhaps just a fragment of it – for an antigen synthesises antigen, which in turn creates an immune response. Already this has been shown to work for influenza (at least in mice) and there are DNA vaccines in the pipeline for herpes, malaria and TB.

Whatever the vector, gene therapy is carried out in one of two ways. In *in vivo* gene therapy, the vector is injected into the body – and has to find its way to the target tissue. The other way is *ex vivo* in which a sample of tissue – tumour cells, for instance – is taken from the patient, treated with the vector and then replaced.

Currently there are around 100 trials of gene therapy underway – more than half of them for cancer. The first ever trial, some years ago now, was on a girl suffering from a rare disorder of the immune system called adenine deaminase (ADA) deficiency. The problem here was simple – just supply a copy of the ADA gene. The treatment worked – but of course not many people have this disease. To be of more general use, we need good clinical results for gene therapy with a disease like cystic fibrosis. Advanced trials are underway but it will be some time before they can be fully evaluated. Meanwhile, some of the gene therapy trials for cancer – done mainly on patients with advanced disease – are showing promising results. For instance, one-third of 60 patients with malignant melanoma experienced shrinkage of their tumours when treated with genes meant to stimulate the immune system.

With gene therapy, it is possible that too much was promised too soon. It is certainly likely to be well into the 21st century before treatments are widely available. And while some optimists still maintain that it will be generally applicable to the whole spectrum of human disease, on current evidence it seem unlikely that this vision will be realised.

Genes, pharmaceuticals and the individual

Most drugs act on proteins – enzymes, receptors or ion channels – as we saw back in Chapter 1. So, in theory, the more proteins we could discover, the more targets there would be for the development of useful drugs. The Human Genome Project (HUGO) is the most powerful way of discovering these new targets. Launched in 1988, under the then leadership of Jim Watson, HUGO aims eventually to discover the entire DNA sequence of the human genome. So far useful maps of the entire genome landscape have been produced, using the latest methods of DNA analysis, which rely – increasingly – upon robots and computers. Hundreds of new genes have been discovered, although only one per cent of the genome has actually been sequenced (however, the technology has been advancing so rapidly that the goal is likely to be achieved sooner rather than later).

Jurgen Drews of the pharmaceutical giant Hoffmann-LaRoche estimates that HUGO will give 3000 to 10,000 new pharmaceutical targets – compared to just 417 which are being studied at the moment. His reasoning goes like this: there are 100 to 150 diseases for which treatments, or improved treatments, are needed. There may be five to ten different genes involved in each, giving 500 to 1000 new targets, once these genes are discovered. And in each disease, there could be from three to ten other proteins which are involved indirectly via biochemical pathways. Put in this multiplier and you arrive at Drew's 3000 to 10,000 figure. New drug targets can also be pinpointed by looking at genes expressed in healthy and diseased states; already research on the genes active in atherosclerotic arteries are yielding interesting results.

It all sounds rather mechanistic – as if humans and their diseases can just be reduced to a specified number of protein targets and drugs developed to hit them. However, there is another way in which HUGO could serve humanity – and one which might not work in the industry's favour if it were fully exploited. As we saw in Chapter 1, people respond very differently to the same drug, and indeed to the same lifestyle measures. It has long been suspected that these individual differences must be genetic in nature, but the technology to tease these out has not been available – until now.

Myriad Genetics, a biotech firm based in Salt Lake City, is developing ways of genotyping humans (in other words, working out their genetic make-up). They have already shown that some people with hypertension have a mutant form of the angiotensinogen gene, which codes for a protein involved in salt regulation. People with this mutation are most likely to benefit from a low salt diet. Similar work at the University of Toronto has pinpointed those schizophrenic patients with a mutation in the dopamine D4 receptor subtype. This group is not likely to benefit from treatment with clozapine. As clozapine is costly and can have severe side effects (as discussed in Chapter 8) this type of knowledge is very valuable to the patient. Where the drug industry could miss out is if this led to individualising the drug to the patient to such an extent that the market for that drug became severely limited.

And finally, HUGO is not the only genome project. Its value has been increased immensely by parallel sequencing of the genomes of many other organisms – the apple, the pig, the common weed *Arabidopsis thaliana* or thale cress, and a number of important pathogens. To date, those which have been completely sequenced are *Mycobacterium tuberculosis* (TB), *Haemophilus influenzae* (meningitis), *Mycobacterium genitalium* (urethitis), *Helicobacter pylori* (gastric ulcer), *Escherichia coli* (food poisoning), and *Borrelia burgdorferi* (Lyme disease). Seqencing projects on *Mycobacterium leprae* (leprosy) and a number of organisms which cause tropical diseases should be completed soon. Finding new drug targets from these genomes could greatly advance the search for new pharmaceutical weapons to fight infectious diseases. And new antibiotics could come from sequencing a *Streptomyces* bacterium. This microbe is not, itself, a pathogen, but is a major source of antibiotics.

A hundred years ago, organic chemistry was on the rise, making the first of the pharmaceutical industry's 'magic molecules'. Into the next millennium, 'magic molecules' will come from a variety of sources – from plants, microbes and marine organisms, if we have the sense to conserve them, and from hi-tech chemical synthesis. With the new genetics we will gain a far better understanding of the enzymes and receptors which are the main drug targets within the body. Together, these two strands of research will ensure that drug molecules reveal more of their 'magic'.

Bibliography

CHAPTER 1

Basic Pharmacology (4th Edition), R. W. Foster, Butterworth Heinemann, 1996.

Medical Pharmacology at a Glance (2nd Edition), M. J. Neal, Blackwell Science, 1992.

Which Medicine: the Essential Consumer Guide to over 1500 Medicines, Rosalind Grant, Consumers Association, 1996.

CHAPTER 2

Plants, People and Culture: the Science of Ethnobotany, Michael J. Balick and Paul Alan Cox, WH Freeman/Scientific American Library, 1996.

Medicinal Chemistry: Principles and Practice, ed. F. D. King, The Royal Society of Chemistry, 1994.

The Principles of Humane Experimental Technique, Rex Burch and William Russell, 1959.

CHAPTER 3

The Virus Hunters: Dispatches from the Front Line, Joseph B. McCormick and Susan Fisher-Hoch, Bloomsbury, 1997.

The Coming Plague: Newly Emerging Diseases in a World out of Balance, Laurie Garrett, Virago, 1994.

Plague's Progress: A Social History of Man and Disease, Arno Karlen, Gollancz, 1995.

Power Unseen: How Microbes Rule the World, Bernard Dixon, W. H. Freeman, 1994.

CHAPTER 4

Raging Hormones: Do They Rule Our Lives?, Gail Vines, Virago, 1993.

Forever Feminine, Robert Wilson.

CHAPTER 6

The Challenge of Pain, Ronald Melzack and Patrick Wall, Penguin, 1988.

CHAPTER 7

Racing to the Beginning of the Road: The Search for the Origins of Cancer, Robert A. Weinberg, Bantam Press, 1997.

CHAPTER 8

Drugs and the Brain, Solomon H. Snyder, Scientific American Library, 1996.

Toxic Psychiatry, Drugs and Electroconvulsive Therapy: The Truth and the Better Alternatives, Peter Breggin, HarperCollins, 1993.

Listening to Prozac: A Psychiatrist Explores Antidepressant Drugs and the Remaking of the Self, Peter D. Kramer, Fourth Estate, 1993.

The Power to Harm: Mind, Murder and Drugs on Trial, John Cornwell, Penguin, 1996.

An Unquiet Mind: A Memoir of Moods and Madness, Kay Redfield Jamison, Picador, 1997.

CHAPTER 9

Buzz: The Science and Lore of Alcohol and Caffeine, Stephen Braun, Oxford University Press, 1996.

To Your Good Health! The Wise Drinkers Guide, Thomas Stuttaford, Faber and Faber, 1977.

Murder, Magic and Medicine, John Mann, Oxford University Press, 1992.

Drugs and Narcotics in History, ed. Roy Porter and Mikuláš Teich, Cambridge University Press, 1995.

Realms of the Human Unconscious, Stanislav Grof.

CHAPTER 10

Nutritional Medicine: the Drug-free Guide to Better Family Health, Stephen Davies and Alan Stewart, Pan, 1987.

The Melatonin Miracle, Walter Pierpaoli and William Rageloon

Melatonin: your Body's Wonder Drug, Russel Reiter and Jo Robinson

CHAPTER 11

The Thread of Life: The Story of Genes and Genetic Engineering, Susan Aldridge, Cambridge University Press, 1996.

Further reading

Science and the Quiet Art: Medical Research and Patient Care, David Weatherall, Oxford University Press, 1995.

The Cambridge Illustrated History of Medicine, ed. Roy Porter, Cambridge University Press, 1996.

The Consumer's Good Chemical Guide: A Jargon-free Guide to the Chemicals of Everyday Life, John Emsley, W. H. Freeman, 1994.

Molecules, P. W. Atkins, Scientific American Library, 1987.

Problem Drugs, Andrew Chetley, Zed Books, 1995.

New Drugs (3rd Edition), ed. John Feely, BMJ, 1994.

Index

Printed in Great
Britain
by Amazon

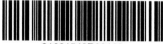